Mechanical Concepts
in
Cardiovascular and Pulmonary
Physiology

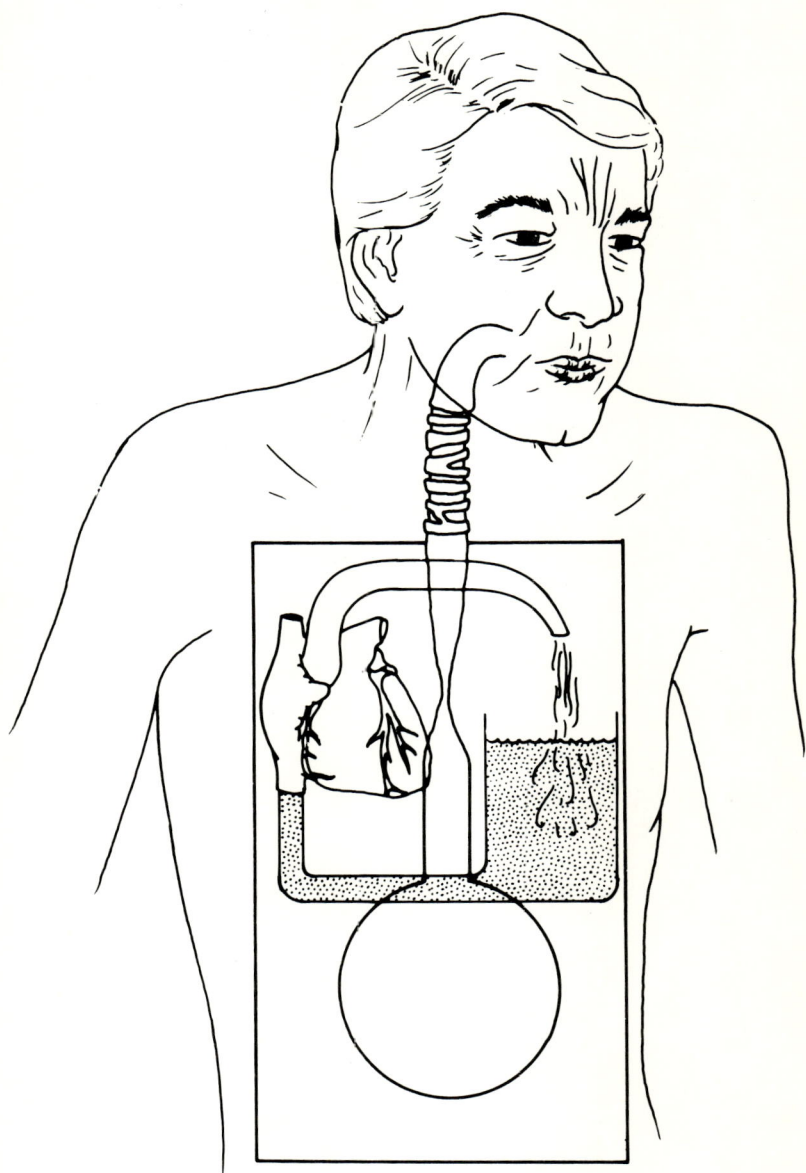

Mechanical Concepts in Cardiovascular and Pulmonary Physiology

JERRY FRANKLIN GREEN, Ph.D.

Assistant Professor of Human Physiology
School of Medicine
University of California
Davis, California

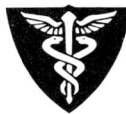

Lea & Febiger • *1977* • *Philadelphia*

Library of Congress Cataloging in Publication Data

Green, Jerry Franklin.
  Mechanical concepts in cardiovascular and pulmonary physiology.

  Bibliography: p.
  Includes index.
  1. Hemodynamics. 2. Lungs. 3. Body fluid flow. 4. Airway
(Medicine) I.   Title. [DNLM: 1.   Cardiovascular   system—
Physiology. 2. Lung—Physiology. 3. Biomechanics. WG102 G796m]
RC105.G73   612'.1181   77-23965
ISBN 0-8121-0598-2

Published in Great Britain by Henry Kimpton Publishers, London

PRINTED IN THE UNITED STATES OF AMERICA

Print number: 4   3   2   1

To Loren Daniel Carlson (1915–1972), *under whose capable guidance many careers were successfully launched. With his long record of fine achievements Dr. Carlson was an inspiration to all with whom he came in contact. He is remembered with deep affection by all who knew him as friend, teacher, and scientific leader.*

Foreword

The time is ripe for a synthesis such as Dr. Green has accomplished in *Mechanical Concepts in Cardiovascular and Pulmonary Physiology*. The title does not convey adequately the beauty of putting the blood vessels and airways into the same conceptual framework. This book exemplifies a recurring phenomenon in science: after a period of elaboration and increasing complexity come unifying concepts with mathematical and graphic models which are both simpler and better predicters of physiological responses than those which were previously available. These advances must be brought together between the covers of a book before they can be easily incorporated into teaching programs and scientific discussions. Dr. Green has performed this latter function in a masterful style. His presentation has evolved from personal teaching experience with medical students and is designed to carry the reader through the fundamentals only. Nevertheless, the list of questions at the end of the book should convince the unwary that a thorough grasp of fundamentals is by no means simple. A student who can understand and answer these questions has the concepts and mathematical skills required for analyzing many of the basic problems related to the mechanics of the cardiovascular and pulmonary systems. These are difficult and often controversial matters. An orderly presentation, emphasizing features which the two systems have in common, is to be hailed.

Baltimore, Maryland RICHARD L. RILEY, M.D.

vii

Preface

Mechanical Concepts in Cardiovascular and Pulmonary Physiology was written for those serious students who wish to obtain a firm conceptual understanding of the physiology of the systemic circulation and of the lung. Through the years numerous textbooks in these fields have been written, all with the same basic approach—discussing structure and function through the presentation of research data. Although an adequate understanding of data is essential for the enlightened physiologist or physician, he must first have an adequate conceptual schema of these systems so that the data may be placed in proper perspective.

Developed in this monograph are schemas of the cardiovascular and pulmonary systems based upon unifying concepts which continually reappear in these systems. For example, the pressure-flow relationships through collapsible tubes describe not only the flow of blood through certain peripheral veins, small arteries and pulmonary capillaries, but also gas flow through the pulmonary airways. Another unifying concept is that of compliance, which describes the pressure-volume relationships of systemic vascular beds, the pulmonary vascular bed, and the pulmonary airways. These basic principles are first discussed in a general fashion and then applied directly to the cardiovascular and pulmonary systems to develop a conceptual schema which will serve the student as a starting point from which to build a deeper understanding of these systems.

It is not the intent of the author to have this volume replace standard textbooks, but to supplement them. *Mechanical Concepts in Cardiovascular and Pulmonary Physiology* was written with students of physiology, medicine, pharmacology, and allied health sciences in mind, and is addressed as well to practicing physicians who desire to develop a firmer understanding of the basic physiology of the cardiovascular and pulmonary systems.

Davis, California   JERRY FRANKLIN GREEN

Acknowledgments

I wish to thank my colleagues who have read early drafts of the manuscript for this text and who have provided their thoughts and criticisms to this book. They include Drs. Walter Ehrlich, Jerry Gillespie, Alan P. Jackman, Glen A. Lillington, Wayne Mitzner, Gibbe Parsons, and Richard L. Riley. I am also grateful to the late Professor Loren D. Carlson who planted the seed for this book. The staff of Lea & Febiger and Mr. George Mundorff, Editor, who have given invaluable help in preparing the manuscript for publication, deserve special commendation. I am also indebted to Jeanne Baldwin for help in typing the manuscript.

J.F.G.

Contents

Contents

SECTION IV: STUDY QUESTIONS

SECTION V: APPENDICES

SECTION 1: MECHANICAL CONCEPTS

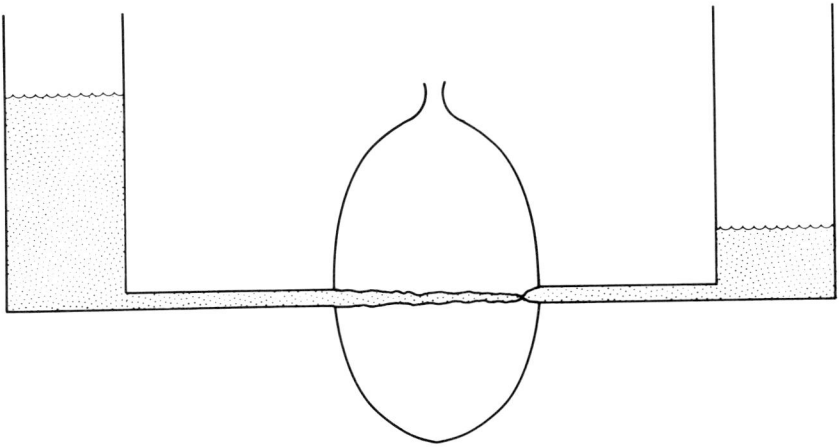

1

Volume-pressure Relationships: The Basics

Numerous elastic structures are found throughout the body: the chest wall, abdominal wall, lungs, urinary bladder, and blood vessels, to mention just a few. The fundamental property of an elastic structure is its inherent ability to offer resistance to a stretching force and to return to its resting or unstressed length or volume after the stretching force has been removed. Elastic elements, such as elastin and collagen within the walls of elastic organs, are responsible for the recoil phenomenon of the organs.

Hooke's law[6] is the basic principle defining elastic behavior; it states that when an elastic substance is stretched a tension develops which is proportional to the degree of deformation which is produced. Hooke's law in its most usual form is applied to longitudinal elements (e.g. a wire or a rubber band) and is expressed by the equation:

$$\frac{F}{A} = Y \frac{L - L_0}{L_0} . \tag{1}$$

The tension developed by stretching is defined as a force per cross-sectional area of the element stretched, F/A (dynes/cm^2); L is the stretched length (cm) and L_0 the resting or "unstressed" length (cm). The quantity Y is the constant of proportionality; it is termed Young's modulus and is a quantitative measure of an element's elasticity.

The term *elasticity* has been interpreted in different ways, and confusion will result unless a single standard definition is used. The proper physical definition of elasticity is "the property of materials which enables them to resist deformation by the development of a resisting force or tension."[6] The popular usage of the term connotes the opposite. If a material is easily stretched (e.g. has a low Young's modulus) it is popularly said to be highly elastic, whereas a material which resists stretch (e. g. has a high Young's modulus) would similarly be regarded as less elastic. As will be shown, the popular concept really refers to the compliance of an elastic object (i.e. its ability to be stretched) rather than to its elasticity in the true sense (i.e. its ability to resist stretch by developing a resistive tension or force).

The confusion between the proper and popular understanding of the term elasticity is so widespread that an author's meaning must be carefully considered. In this volume the physical definition of elasticity is used. Thus, if Y is high relative to some normal value, the element would resist stretch easily and be considered to be less elastic. A steel wire would have a high Young's modulus whereas a rubber band would have a low one. Figure 1 illustrates the relationship which is defined by Hooke's law.

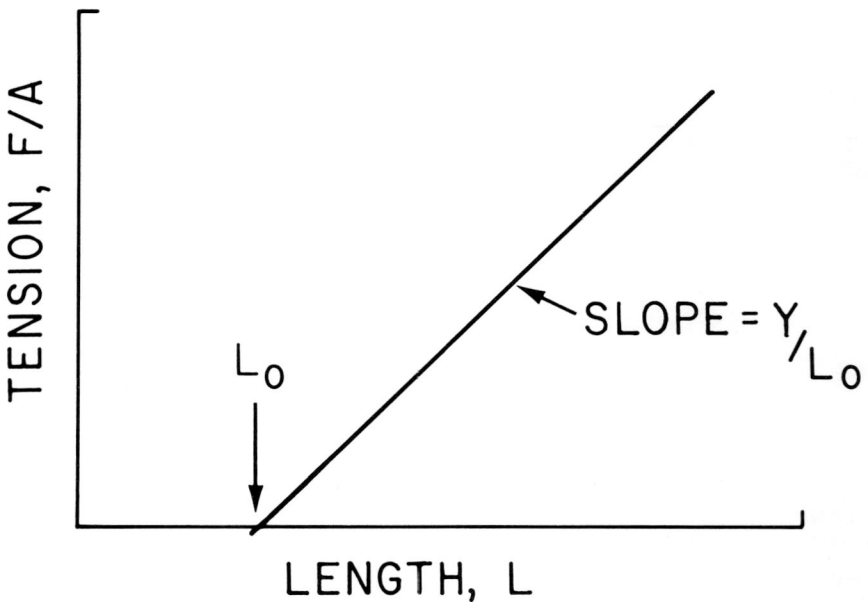

Fig. 1.   Length-tension relationship of an elastic element as defined by Hooke's law.

Since Hooke's law has to be applied to longitudinal elements, it is difficult for most physiologists to use this relationship to define elastic behavior of anatomic structures simply because most such structures are not longitudinal elements but more akin to sacs (i.e. the lung) or cylinders (i.e. the blood vessels). Some physiologists investigating elastic behavior of certain selected blood vessels have worked around this problem by cutting helical strips of vessel and measuring the length-tension relationship of these strips, but this approach has limited applicability.[2,29,15,30] It is misleading to cut a lung into strips to investigate its elastic behavior, which partly derives from its sac-like structure.

Physiologists, therefore, have found it more useful to quantitate the degree of elasticity of an anatomic structure by measuring the change in volume of the structure which results from a given distending pressure. To illustrate this principle, let us consider the case of the three elastic balloons pictured in Figure 2. The coiled lines around the balloons represent the elastic elements within the walls. The arrows represent the degree of recoil produced by the elastic elements, i.e. the speed with which the balloons will collapse when the distending force is withdrawn. The pressure distending each balloon is the difference between the pressure within the balloon and the pressure

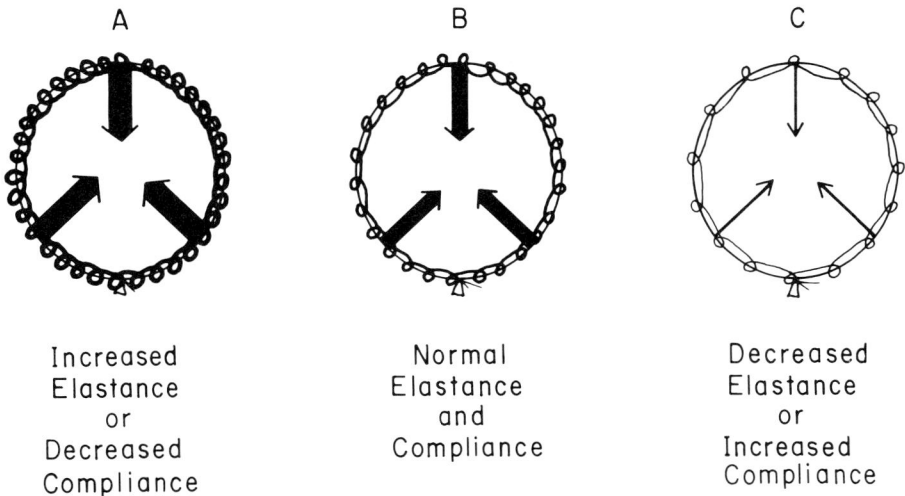

A	B	C
Increased Elastance or Decreased Compliance	Normal Elastance and Compliance	Decreased Elastance or Increased Compliance

Fig. 2.   Hypothetical balloons possessing different elastic content.

outside the balloon and is called the *transmural pressure*, symbolized by P_{TM}. Thus,

$$P_{TM} = \text{transmural pressure} = P_{inside} - P_{outside} \, .$$

This is a basic relationship which will be discussed in more detail later in the text.

Even though the volume of each balloon in Figure 2 is the same, the transmural pressure in each is markedly different. Thus, the transmural pressure in balloon A is greater than that of balloon B, and the transmural pressure in balloon C is less than that of balloon B. This is true because there is a greater amount of elastic substance within the wall of balloon A, causing a greater inward-acting recoil force and, therefore, requiring a greater internal pressure to maintain the same degree of distension. In contrast, the lesser amount of elastic substance in balloon C results in a lesser recoil force. It would appear from this example that to quantitate the elasticity of an elastic structure we would need to know the distending pressure and the absolute volume of the structure; to compare the elasticities of different structures, we need only adjust the volume of each structure to obtain some given volume (the same for all structures) and note the different distending pressure. This procedure would be difficult to carry out for most physiologic systems. The desired information, however, could be obtained by simply changing the volume and observing the changes in pressure. The ratio of the change in pressure to change in volume, i.e. the slope of the volume-pressure curve, is called the *elastance* and serves as a quantitative measure of the elasticity of the structure in question. We do not need to know the absolute values but only the relative changes of these parameters.

Although the term elastance is extremely descriptive, i.e. an increased elastance means greater elasticity, most physiologists prefer to define elastic behavior in terms of *compliance*. Compliance is nothing more than the reciprocal of elastance and can thus be defined as:

$$C = \frac{\Delta V}{\Delta P} \, , \tag{2}$$

where C = compliance, $\triangle V$ = change in volume, and $\triangle P$ = change in transmural pressure.

To summarize what has been said thus far we may state that elastance is an index of the ability of a structure to resist deformation by stress, whereas compliance describes the ability of a structure to give way (undergo deformation) by a stress. An easily inflatable balloon has high compliance and low elastance, whereas a stiff balloon which strongly resists inflation has a low compliance and high elastance.

Figure 3 illustrates the volume-pressure relationships we would obtain from the balloons pictured in Figure 2. Notice that the slope of the volume-pressure curve for balloon A is much steeper than that for the other balloons, indicating that for a given change in volume a greater pressure results. This is exactly what would be expected considering the greater elasticity in balloon A. Balloon A is thus "stiff" relative to normal (balloon B) and has decreased compliance, whereas balloon C is "flabby" relative to normal and has increased compliance.*

Although compliance is usually defined as the ratio of the change in volume to the change in pressure, a more specific definition is often needed.[19,17,8] Thus,

$$C = \frac{V - V_0}{P - O} \; , \tag{3}$$

where V_0 is the resting or *unstressed volume*, i.e. the volume contained within the compliant structure when the pressure, P, within the compliant structure is zero (0), and V is the volume *above* the unstressed volume. The above relationship is demonstrated in Figure 4. Notice the similarity between this figure and Figure 1, which illustrates the relationship defined by Hooke's law. The unstressed volume (V_0) is analogous to the unstressed length (L_0), the reciprocal of the compliance coefficient ($1/C$) is analogous to Y/L_0, and pressure is analogous to tension. Thus even though it may be difficult or even impossible to quantitate the elastic properties of an anatomic structure by measuring the length-tension relationships, the same kind of

---

*Note that the concept of compliance avoids much of the confusion produced by the terms elasticity and elastance. For this reason it is to be preferred.

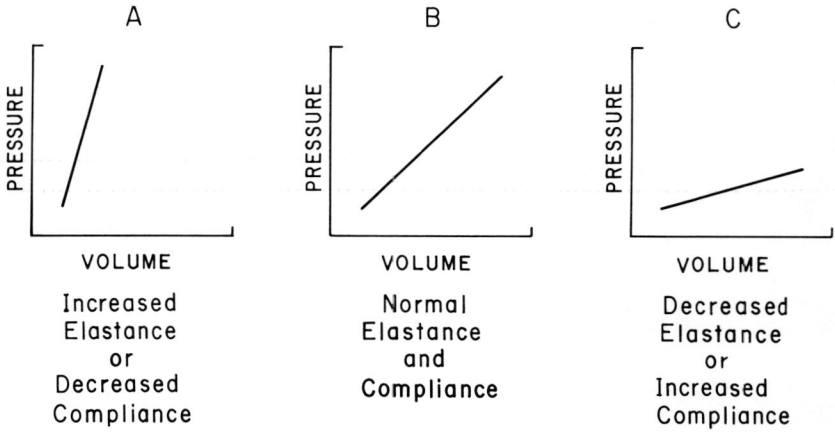

A	B	C
Increased Elastance or Decreased Compliance	Normal Elastance and Compliance	Decreased Elastance or Increased Compliance

Fig. 3. Volume-pressure relationships of the balloons illustrated in Figure 2.

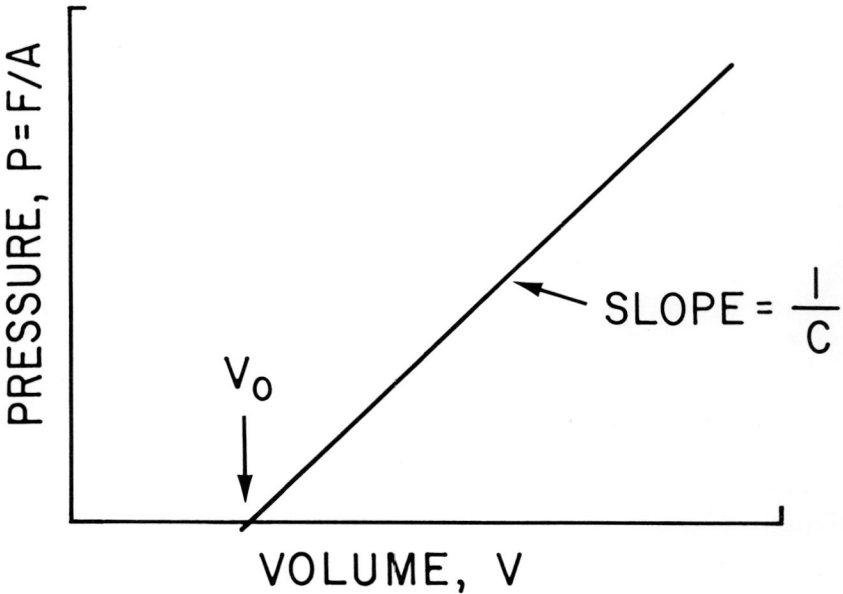

Fig. 4. Graphic solution of Equation 3 illustrating how the volume-pressure relationship of an elastic structure is analogous to the length-tension relationship defined by Hooke's law (Eq. 1) and illustrated in Figure 1.

information may be obtained by measuring the volume-pressure relationships and using the compliance as an index of elasticity.

The units of pressure used by most physiologists are cm H_2O or mm Hg; therefore compliance is most often expressed as ml/cm H_2O or ml/mm Hg. Since 1 cm H_2O = 0.738 mm Hg, the above units may be interconverted by multiplying ml/cm H_2O by 1/0.738 or ml/mm Hg by 1/1.355. Volume is frequently normalized on the basis of body weight; thus we can find compliance expressed as $ml \cdot kg^{-1} \cdot mm\ Hg^{-1}$.

In summary, the relationship of volume to pressure is a useful method of measuring the inherent elasticity of a distensible structure.

2

Pressure-flow Relationships: The Basics

The physical principles which govern the flow of fluids through conducting passages, i.e. vessels and airways, whether rigid or collapsible, are derived from the general laws of hydrodynamics.[41] The fluid may be either liquid, such as blood flowing through the cardiovascular system, or air such as we breathe. The difference in these fluids lies in their different densities and viscosities. This chapter on pressure-flow relationships contains a discussion of flow through rigid tubes followed by a discussion of flow through collapsible tubes. In these discussions the fluid will be considered a liquid, yet the principles would be the same for air flow.

FLOW THROUGH RIGID TUBES

The basic expression for the flow of fluid through rigid tubes is that of Poiseuille's law, which states that the volume of fluid flowing past a point in the tube per unit time ($\dot{Q}$) is proportional to the difference in pressure between the inflow and outflow end of the tube ($P_1 - P_0$) and the fourth power of the radius (r) of the tube, and inversely proportional to the length of the tube (l) and viscosity of the fluid (η). (A derivation of Poiseuille's law, with certain other basic laws of hydrodynamics, may be found in Appendix II.)

In mathematical terms Poiseuille's law may be expressed as follows for conditions of horizontal flow:

$$\frac{P_I - P_O}{\dot{Q}} = \frac{8\eta L}{\pi r^4} = R. \qquad (4)$$

The quantity $\frac{8\eta L}{\pi r^4}$ represents those factors which tend to retard flow and is referred to as the resistance to flow, R. The ratio of the difference in driving pressure to flow is used as an empirical way of defining the resistance to flow. Since in most physiologic systems l and η remain constant, a change in R is interpreted as a change in the radius of the tube (i.e. blood vessel or airway). The unit for resistance in the centimeter-gram-second (cgs) system is dynes·sec/cm^5, pressure being expressed as dynes/cm^2 and flow as cm^3/sec. Since in practice pressure is measured as mm Hg and flow as L/min, resistance is usually expressed as mm Hg per L/min (mm Hg·L^{-1}·min).

The most commonly used form of the Poiseuille equation is obtained by rearranging Equation 4 as follows:

$$\dot{Q} = \frac{1}{R}(P_I - P_O). \qquad (5)$$

Two possible ways of graphically displaying Equation 5 are presented in Figure 5. Horizontal flow is assumed. The slope of the pressure-flow curve is equal to the reciprocal of the resistance (1/R); the steeper the slope, the less the resistance. The linearity of the pressure-flow relationship derived from Poiseuille's law implies constant radius, length, viscosity, and laminar flow (see Appendix II). The pressure surrounding a rigid tube has no effect on the pressure-flow relationship; this is, however, not the case with a collapsible tube, as will be shown.

FLOW THROUGH COLLAPSIBLE TUBES—
THE HYDRODYNAMICS OF STARLING RESISTORS

An ideal collapsible tube is any tube made of material with characteristics such that any finite positive transmural pressure causes it to be fully open and any finite negative transmural pressure (at the outflow end) causes it to collapse (at the outflow end). The pressure-flow relationships of such a tube are governed primarily by Poiseuille's law under conditions where the tube has a positive transmural pressure throughout, i.e. flow is propor-

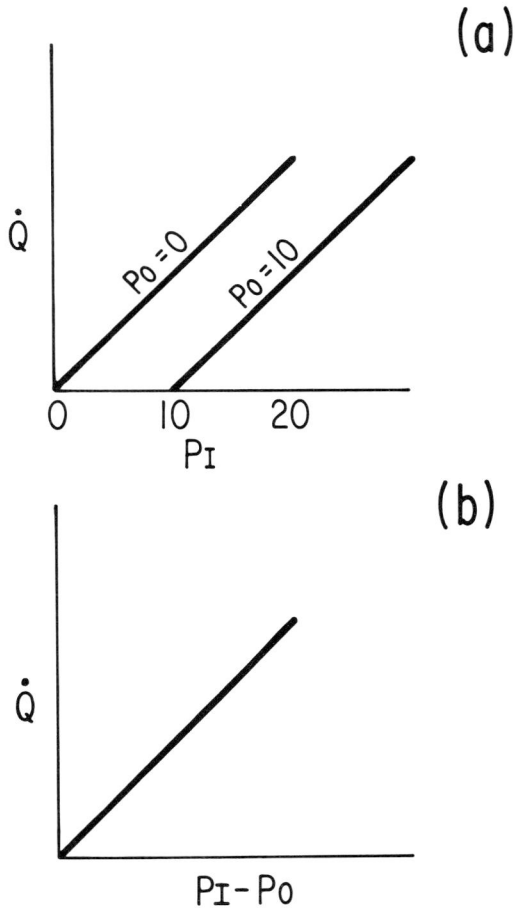

Fig. 5. Pressure-flow relationships for a rigid horizontal tube. The zero reference point for pressure is taken at the level of the tube. a: Pressure-flow relationships obtained with two different outflow pressures (P_0) when flow ($\dot{Q}$) is plotted as a function of inflow pressure (P_I). b: Pressure-flow relationship obtained for all outflow pressures when flow is plotted as a function of the driving pressure ($P_I - P_0$). This figure assumes the resistance is independent of pressures. Note the invariance of the slope (characteristic of the tube and viscosity of fluid) and the fact that the pressure surrounding the tube is irrelevant (compare with Fig. 8).

tional to the difference between the inflow and outflow pressure, and the pressure surrounding the tube has no effect upon flow. Under conditions where a finite negative transmural pressure develops at the outflow end, the tube becomes partially constricted (collapsed) at the outflow end, and the pressure surrounding the tube becomes most significant because it now replaces the outflow pressure as the back pressure to perfusion. A schematic drawing of an ideal collapsible tube (Starling resistor) is presented in Figure 6.* In this illustration the pressure at the outflow end of the tube (P_O) is equal to atmospheric pressure. Since the pressure surrounding the tube (P_S) is greater than P_O, flow is proportional to the difference between the inflow pressure (P_I) and (P_S), i.e. $\dot{Q} \propto P_I - P_S$. The resistance to flow, at constant viscosity, is a function of the length and diameter of the tube up to, but not including, the area of collapse.

The pressure-flow relationships through an ideal Starling resistor may be succinctly summarized by the following three statements: (1) Whenever the surrounding pressure is greater

---

*Knowlton and Starling[23] first used such a device in their heart-lung preparation as a means of controlling "peripheral resistance." They employed a thin-walled collapsible tube, traversing a chamber. The pressure in the chamber surrounding the tube could be set at any desired level. Since the time of Starling, whenever a collapsible tube has been used in this manner, it has been known as a Starling resistor. Although the Starling resistor has been widely used in physiologic laboratories since the time of Starling, it was not until 1941 that quantitative studies of the pressure-flow relationships through such tubes were undertaken and the physiologic significance of these relationships was recognized. Holt,[20] studying flow through collapsible tubes, found that lowering the outflow pressure did not significantly change flow when the outflow pressure was less than the pressure surrounding the collapsible segment of the tube. Reasoning from this model he concluded that the collapse of veins as they entered the chest accounted for the fact that atrial pressure may change independently of a change in peripheral venous pressure. In a theoretical discussion of energy and hydraulic gradients along systemic veins, based on a model of flow through collapsible tubes, Duomarco and Rimini[12] pointed out an unusual independence of flow and pressure; this accounts for the reason negative intrathoracic pressure does not directly alter venous return. Rodbard[31] compared the pressure-flow relationships of a rigid tube with a collapsible Penrose tube of the same dimensions. He demonstrated that the flow was markedly influenced by the pressure surrounding the collapsible tube, and that the addition of an outflow resistance when the tube was collapsed had no influence on flow. He suggested that the special dynamics of collapsible tubes may account for certain paradoxical findings in flow through partially stenosed vessels.

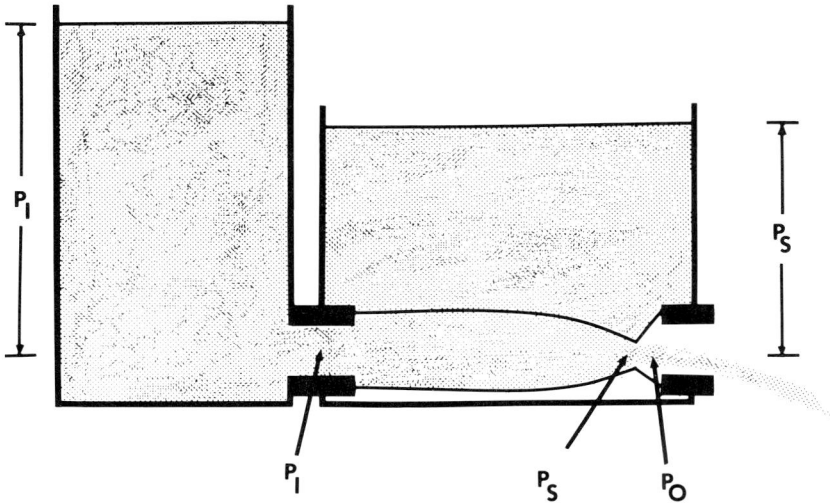

Fig. 6. Schematic drawing of an ideal Starling resistor. P_I = inflow pressure, P_S = surrounding pressure, and P_O = outflow pressure = atmospheric pressure. Flow is proportional to the difference between the inflow pressure and the surrounding pressure.

than the inflow pressure no flow occurs through the tube. (2) Whenever inflow pressure is greater than surrounding pressure and surrounding pressure is greater than outflow pressure, flow is proportional to the difference between inflow pressure and surrounding pressure, and changes in outflow pressure have no influence on flow. (3) Whenever inflow pressure is greater than outflow pressure and outflow pressure is greater than surrounding pressure, flow is proportional to the difference between inflow pressure and outflow pressure, and changes in surrounding pressure have no influence on flow. The three possible conditions of a Starling resistor are depicted in Figure 7 as hydraulic models.

An intuitive understanding as to why P_S functions as a back pressure to perfusion under conditions where $P_S > P_O$ may be obtained by considering what happens at the downstream end of a Starling resistor. The pressure at the downstream end* can never deviate significantly above or below P_S. If it did rise above

---

*The downstream end of the Starling resistor refers to the area of collapse. The outflow pressure is the pressure distal to the area of collapse.

Condition 1

$$P_S > P_I > P_O$$
$$\dot{Q} = 0$$

Condition 2

$$P_I > P_S > P_O$$
$$\dot{Q} \propto P_I - P_S$$
$$P_O \quad \text{irrelevant}$$

Condition 3

$$P_I > P_O > P_S$$
$$\dot{Q} \propto P_I - P_O$$
$$P_S \quad \text{irrelevant}$$

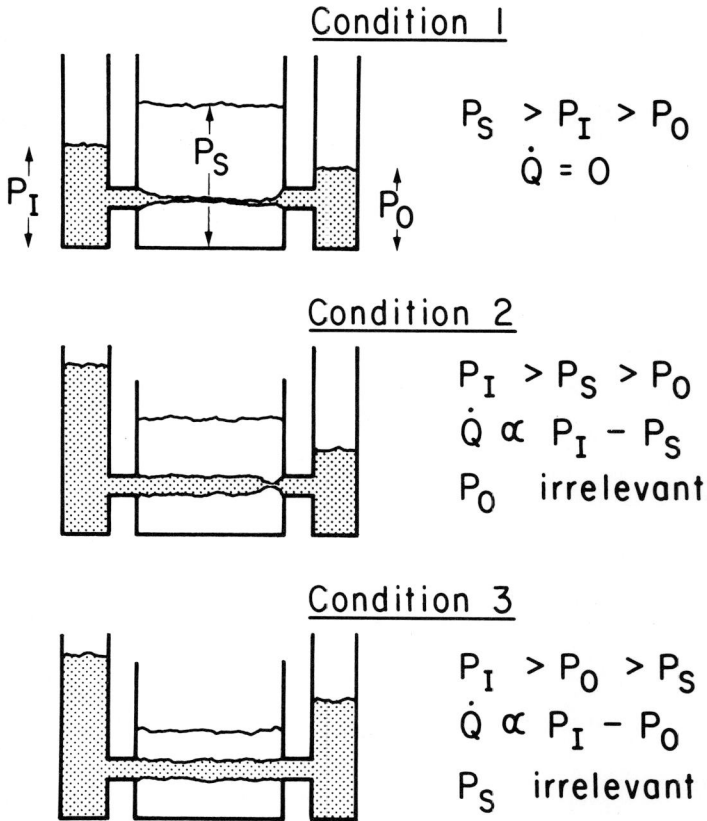

Fig. 7. Hydraulic models depicting the three conditions of a Starling resistor. (From Green, J. F.: The pulmonary circulation. In: *The Peripheral Circulations* (R. Zelis, Ed.). New York, Grune & Stratton, 1975. Reproduced here with permission of the publishers.)

P_S the tube would be wide open, and the pressure would then be dissipated into the lower pressure system at the outflow end of the tube (P_O). If the pressure at the downstream end of the tube were less than P_S, the tube would shut completely and flow would cease. Thus, pressure at the downstream end of an ideal Starling resistor becomes equal to P_S and independent of flow and, as such, functions as a *pressure load* and not a resistance (resistance being related according to Poiseuille's law, at constant viscosity, to the length and diameter of the tube upstream from the point where P_S acts). For this reason P_S becomes the back pressure to perfusion whenever $P_I > P_S > P_O$; hence:

$$\dot{Q} = \frac{1}{R} (P_I - P_S) .\tag{6}$$

Changing P_O would have no influence on $\dot{Q}$ unless $P_O \geq P_S$. If this occurred, the transmural pressure at the distal end of the tube would become positive, the tube would open, and P_O would replace P_S in the above equation for it would then be the back pressure. Similarly, a change in flow would have no influence on P_O when $P_S \geq P_O$. These unusual relationships, where a change in flow has no influence in the pressure drop across the outflow constriction ($P_S - P_O$), and a change in this pressure drop has no influence on flow, are accomplished by the automatic control of the cross-sectional area of the outflow constriction as described by Permutt and Riley.[28] It should be emphasized that P_S acts as a pressure load and not a resistance. Thus, the term "Starling resistor" is actually a misnomer. Misinterpretation of this critical point can lead to much confusion. The pressure-flow relationships of Starling resistors are plotted in various ways in Figure 8. The three examples presented were chosen because they are identical to the pressure-flow relationships obtained in different physiologic systems: the pulmonary airway, the pulmonary circulation, the systemic arteries, and the systemic veins. All three relationships will again be met in later chapters. Careful study and thought about this figure will assure the reader of a complete understanding of the hydrodynamics of collapsible tubes.

In summary, when a collapsible tube is surrounded by a pressure which is greater than its outflow pressure, it will collapse at its distal end, a change in flow will have no influence on the pressure drop across the constricted end of the tube, and a change in pressure drop across the end of the tube will have no influence on flow, flow being determined only by Equation 6. The physiologic significance of these relationships comes from the fact that many areas of the cardiovascular and pulmonary systems behave analogously to Starling resistors.

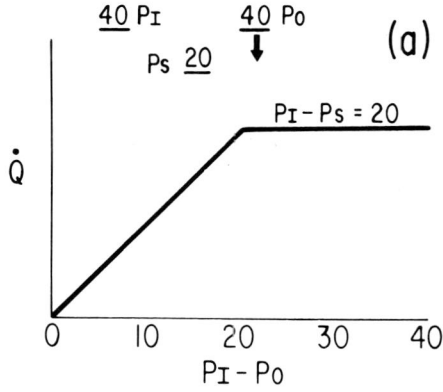

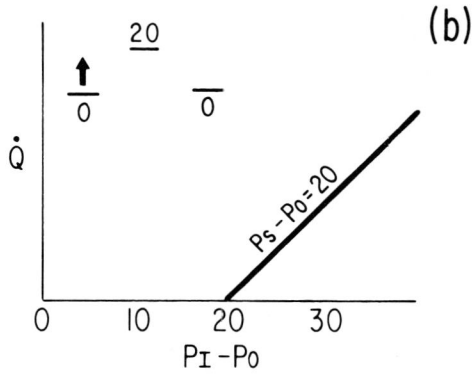

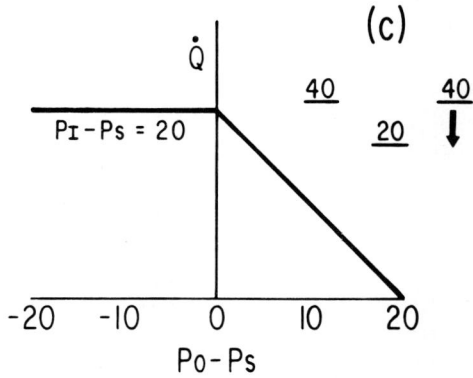

MEANING OF RESISTANCE

In most physiologic systems an increase in the resistance to flow, calculated as the ratio of the driving pressure to flow, is generally interpreted as a decrease in the radius of the conduit(s) through which the flow is occurring, since the length and viscosity tend to remain constant. Although this is an accurate interpretation under most conditions, there are situations where an increase in the resistance ratio should best be interpreted simply as an indication that an increased amount of potential energy has been dissipated somewhere throughout the flow circuit. A classical example of such a situation may be found in the pulmonary vascular bed. As we shall discuss in a later chapter, the pulmonary capillaries are believed to function as Starling resistors. That is, whenever the alveolar pressure (the pressure surrounding the pulmonary capillaries) is greater than the pulmonary venous pressure (outflow pressure), the pressure at the outflow end of the pulmonary capillaries becomes equal to alveolar pressure and alveolar pressure functions as the back pressure. Whenever alveolar pressure rises, as with positive

---

Fig. 8. Pressure-flow relationships for a thin-walled horizontal collapsible tube. The zero reference point for pressures is taken at the level of the tube. Note the invariance of the slope (characteristic of the tube and viscosity of the fluid) and the fact that the surrounding pressure (P_S) is not irrelevant. The inserts represent the relative levels of P_I, P_S, and P_O. a: The pressure-flow relationship obtained when flow ($\dot{Q}$) is plotted as a function of the difference between inflow (P_I) and outflow (P_O) pressures. The example is given for $P_I = P_O = 40$ and $P_S = 20$. As P_O is lowered at constant P_I and P_S, $\dot{Q}$ increases until P_O becomes equal to P_S ($P_I - P_O = P_I - P_S$). As P_O is lowered below P_S, P_S becomes the effective back pressure and flow remains constant. Once $P_O \leq P_S$, $\dot{Q}$ is unaffected by P_O. b: The pressure-flow relationship obtained when $\dot{Q}$, as in (a), is plotted as a function of $P_I - P_O$; however, in this example $P_I = P_O = 0$, $P_S = 20$, and the pressure-flow relationship is obtained by raising P_I at constant P_S and P_O. As P_I is raised no flow occurs until P_I exceeds P_S ($P_I - P_O = P_S - P_O$); thereafter $\dot{Q}$ increases as P_I exceeds P_S. Again, changes in P_O have no effect on $\dot{Q}$ as long as $P_O \leq P_S$. Note that with the Starling resistor different types of pressure-flow relationships can be obtained by either lowering P_O at constant P_I and P_S or by raising P_I at constant P_O and P_S. This is to be contrasted with the rigid system where the same relationship (Fig. 5) is obtained by either raising P_I or lowering P_O at constant (and irrelevant) P_S. c: The pressure-flow relationship obtained when $\dot{Q}$ is plotted as a function of $P_O - P_S$. In this example as in example (a) $P_I = P_O = 40$ and $P_S = 20$. As P_O is lowered (decreasing $P_O - P_S$) $\dot{Q}$ increases until $P_O \leq P_S$ $P_I - P_O = P_I - P_S$); thereafter $\dot{Q}$ remains constant because the driving pressure $P_I - P_S$ is constant. Again changes in P_O, when $P_O \leq P_S$, have no effect on $\dot{Q}$.

pressure ventilation, pulmonary vascular resistance, calculated as the difference between pulmonary arterial and left atrial pressure divided by cardiac output, also rises. Since the increase in alveolar pressure functions as an increased pressure load and not an increased resistance, the increase in the calculated pulmonary vascular resistance results from an increased dissipation of energy across the downstream end of the pulmonary capillaries and does not reflect changes in the upstream dimensions of the vessel or viscosity of the blood. Therefore, before an adequate interpretation of resistance measurements ($\triangle P/\triangle \dot{Q}$) can be made, the investigator must be keenly aware of the type of system that is being measured (rigid versus collapsible) and the effective back pressure used in the resistance equation.

EFFECT OF GRAVITY ON PRESSURE-FLOW RELATIONSHIPS

Until now we have been careful to discuss pressure-flow relationships for rigid and collapsible systems under conditions of horizontal flow. Under nonhorizontal conditions hydrostatic factors affect the pressure-flow relationship, although if the basic hydrodynamics of horizontal flow are thoroughly understood there should be no problem in understanding the effect of gravity. When a flow system (either rigid or collapsible) is tilted in a gravitational field, the upstream driving pressure (P_I) is modified relative to the back pressure by the resulting hydrostatic pressure effect, ρgh, where ρ is the density of the fluid, g is the magnitude of the gravitational or acceleration stress, h is the difference in levels between the inflow segment of the flow system and the point in the system where the back pressure is manifest. To introduce hydrostatic effects, an effective inflow pressure, $P_{I\ eff}$, must replace P_I in all flow equations, where:

$$P_{I\ eff} = P_I \pm \rho gh. \tag{7}$$

When the inflow pressure is at a higher horizontal level than the back pressure, $P_{I\ eff} = P_I + \rho gh$, and when the inflow pressure is at a lower horizontal level than the back pressure, $P_{I\ eff} = P_I - \rho gh$.
Substituting Equation 7 in Equations 5 and 6 yields:

$$\dot{Q} = \frac{(P_I \pm \rho gh) - P_0}{R}, \tag{8}$$

for rigid systems and

$$\dot{Q} = \frac{(P_I \pm \rho gh) - P_S}{R},$$ (9)

for collapsible systems.

Gravity has a profound effect upon the cardiovascular system. This will be discussed in Chapter 5. Figure 9 illustrates schematically the effect of gravity on a rigid flow system.

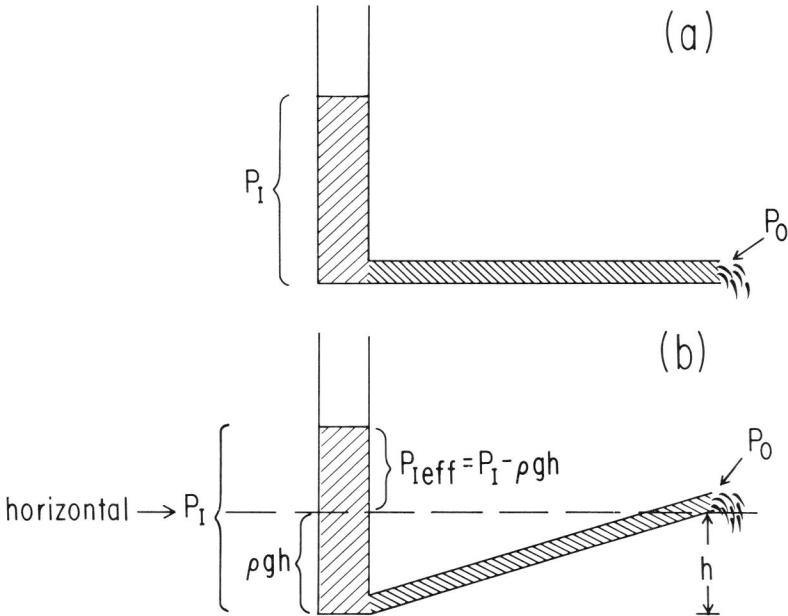

Fig. 9. Hydraulic model illustrating the effect of gravity on a rigid flow system. *a:* In the horizontal plane, flow ($\dot{Q}$) is proportional to the inflow (P_I) and the outflow (P_O) pressures. *b:* If the inflow reservoir is lowered relative to the system's outflow, the effective inflow pressure ($P_{I\ eff}$) is reduced by an amount (ρgh) proportional to the distance the reservoir was lowered (h). To say it another way, the volume in the reservoir below the level of the outflow does not partake in the generation of a flow gradient.

SECTION II: CIRCULATORY MECHANICS

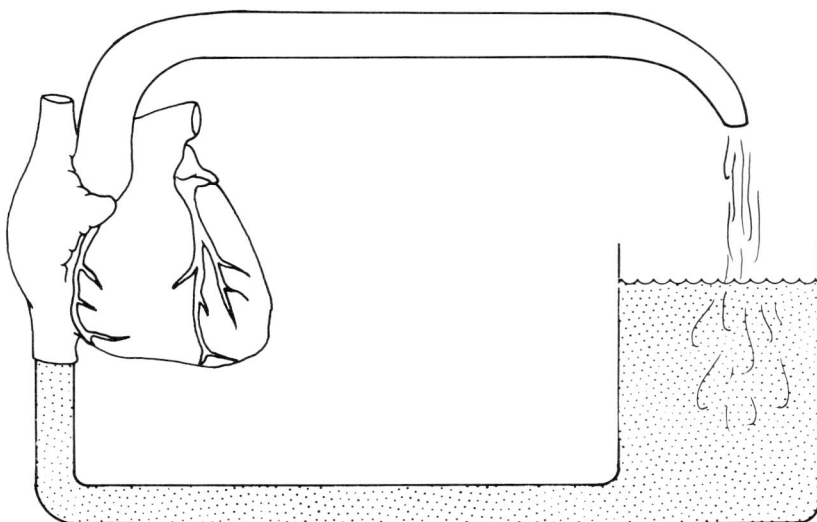

3

Volume-pressure Relationships of the Circulatory System

Systemic and pulmonary blood vessels are elastic structures. This is demonstrated by their inherent ability to recoil after a deformation-producing stress has been removed. In the intact body the deforming stress is an increase in the intravascular fluid volume. Such increases in the vascular volume will stretch the walls of the vessels and the recoil of the elastic vessel walls will increase the intravascular pressure. The relationship of vascular volume to vascular transmural pressure is called *vascular compliance*, and measures the inherent elasticity of the vascular system in much the same way as alveolar compliance measures lung elasticity (Chap. 10).

SYSTEMIC VASCULAR COMPLIANCE

The total lumped compliance of the systemic circulation * can be measured in experimental animals by momentarily stopping the circulation (usually by electrically fibrillating the ventricles) and rapidly equalizing the arterial and venous pressures by pumping blood from arteries to veins.[19] The intravascular pressure which is measured when arterial and venous pressures are equal is the static transmural pressure of the system at that blood volume and is called the *mean systemic pressure* (P_{MS}). The circulation is reestablished by an electrical shock to the heart,

---

*The term *lumped systemic compliance* simply treats conceptually the compliances of the arteries, capillaries, and veins as a single compliance.

Table 1.   Reported Values for Systemic Arterial, Lumped Systemic, and Lumped Pulmonary Compliance

Compliance Value	Reference
Systemic arterial	
0.067 ml·kg^{-1}·mm Hg^{-1}	35
Lumped systemic (systemic venous)	
1.4 ml·kg^{-1}·mm Hg^{-1}	19
1.8 ml·kg^{-1}·mm Hg^{-1}	8
2.3 ml·kg^{-1}·mm Hg^{-1}	33
2.4 ml·kg^{-1}·mm Hg^{-1}	34
3.3 ml·kg^{-1}·mm Hg^{-1}	16
4.2 ml·kg^{-1}·mm Hg^{-1}	11
2.57 (average)	
Lumped pulmonary	
.217 ml·kg^{-1}·mm Hg^{-1}	19
.213 ml·kg^{-1}·mm Hg^{-1}	13
.366–.627 ml·kg^{-1}·mm Hg	25

and the total blood volume is increased by a known amount. The mean systemic pressure is again measured by the stop-flow procedure. The ratio of the change in volume to change in mean systemic pressure is the lumped compliance of the systemic circulation, C_S. Values of C_S in the dog have ranged from 1.4 to 4.2 ml·kg^{-1}·mm Hg^{-1} (Table 1).

Independent measurements of arterial compliance, C_a, of the dog have been measured as 0.067 ml·kg^{-1}·mm Hg^{-1} by rapidly removing a known quantity of blood from the arterial system at constant cardiac output and recording the fall in arterial pressure.[35] C_a is, thus, 30 to 60 times less than C_S. Because the compliance of the arterial system is so small compared with the compliance of the total systemic circulation, the venous compliance, C_V, is considered as a first approximation to be equal to C_S.

The relative differences between systemic arterial and venous compliances are graphically illustrated by their respective volume-pressure curves; these are seen in Figure 10 and were drawn from reported values for both arterial and venous compliances as presented in Table 1. None of theses values, obviously, is entirely correct; the range can probably be accounted for by experimental error and the slight difference in

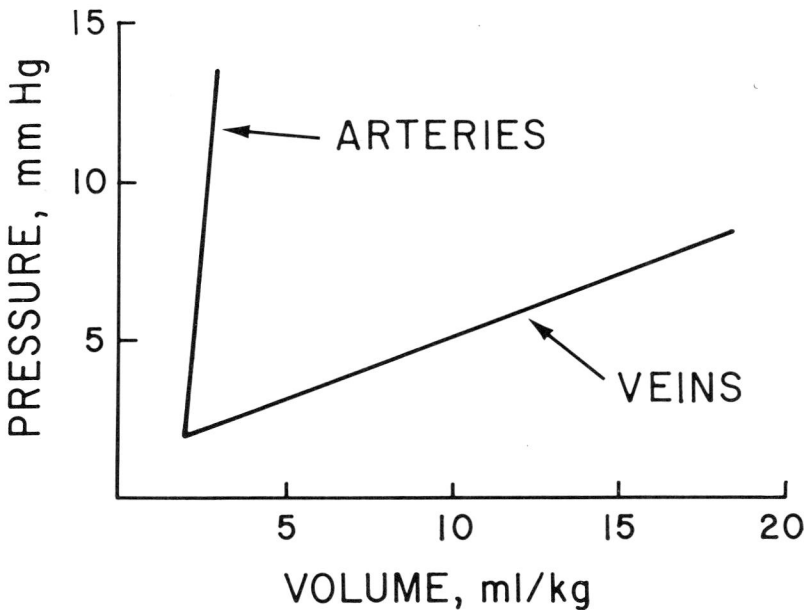

Fig. 10.   Volume-pressure curves of the systemic arterial and venous systems. These curves were drawn from the average data presented in Table 1. A given change in volume results in a much smaller change in venous pressure than in arterial pressure because of a greater venous compliance.

the techniques used to measure them. What is important about the values presented in Table 1 is that they demonstrate relative differences between venous and arterial compliances in the systemic circulation. Consider the following example: If 100 ml of blood were rapidly injected into the arterial system of a 70-kg man (assuming compliance values presented in Table 1) the arterial pressure would rise approximately 21 mm Hg; however, if that same volume was rapidly injected into the venous system, the venous pressure would rise less than 1 mm Hg. This basic difference in the volume-pressure relationship of the arterial and venous systems, which is related to anatomic differences in these two basic types of vessels, has a profound influence on overall circulatory mechanics.

PULMONARY VASCULAR COMPLIANCE

Pulmonary vessels, like those in the systemic circulation, are elastic; however, their compliance is quantitatively different.

Historically the pulmonary circulation has been considered a highly distensible system. When the basis for this conclusion is analyzed, we find that most authors mean that the pulmonary arterial system (usually the pulmonary artery) is more compliant than the systemic arterial system (usually the aorta). Yet, when the lumped compliance of the pulmonary system (arteries, capillaries, and veins) is compared to the lumped compliance of the systemic system, the pulmonary system is found to be significantly less compliant than that of the systemic bed. The lumped compliance of the pulmonary vascular bed has been measured in the dog and found to be 0.217 ml·kg^{-1}·mm Hg^{-1}.[19] Thus, for an average 12-kg dog under static conditions (i.e. when the circulation has been stopped and pressures throughout the pulmonary vascular bed have been equalized) an increase in volume of 2.6 ml will cause the pressure to rise 1 mm Hg. This value for the compliance of the whole pulmonary vascular bed is substantially lower than the compliance values reported for the entire systemic vascular bed (Table 1). Other studies of pulmonary vascular compliance have yielded similar values.

The relative differences in the compliance of the systemic and pulmonary vascular beds is most dramatically illustrated by comparing their respective volume-pressure curves in Figure 11.

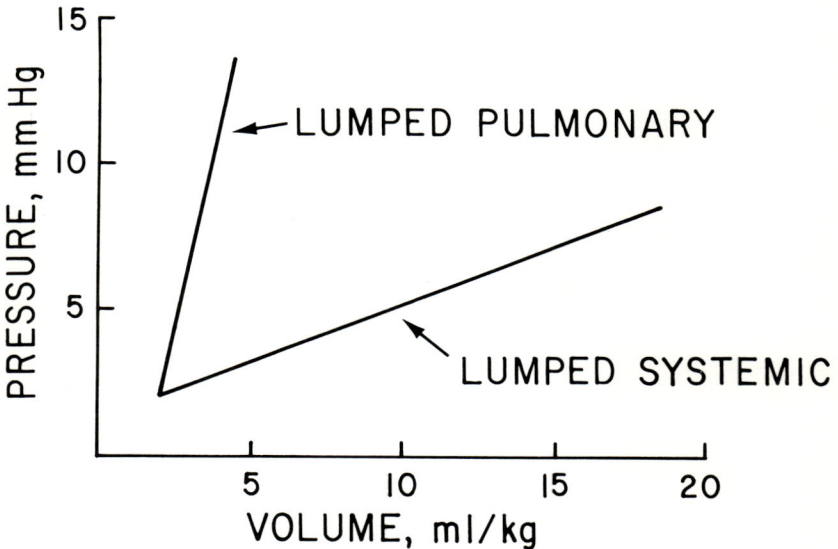

Fig. 11.   Volume-pressure curves of the systemic and pulmonary vascular beds. These curves were drawn from the data presented in Table 1.

The systemic curve was drawn from the average compliance calculated from the data presented in Table 1.

The compliance of the serial sections of the pulmonary vascular bed is distributed somewhat like that in the systemic circulation. The compliances of large pulmonary artery and vein were found to be about equal, each accounting for about 15 percent of the total pulmonary vascular compliance. The small pulmonary vessels, small veins, venules, and capillaries account for the rest of the pulmonary vascular compliance.[13]

In summary, the blood vessels of both the systemic and pulmonary circulations are elastic structures and, as such, recoil inward when a volume stress is applied. The total compliance of the systemic circulation is greater than that of the pulmonary circulation, and the venous systems of both circulations possess the greatest compliance. The functional significance of these volume-pressure relationships will be discussed in the next chapter.

4

A Conceptual Model of the
Circulatory System

In this chapter we will develop a conceptual schema of the circulatory system, which can then be used as a framework upon which to hang much of the minutia (gee-whiz numbers) presented in this and other textbooks of physiology. For the purpose of simplicity, the coronary and bronchial circulations are not considered.

The cardiovascular system can be conceptually broken down into two major subdivisions: (1) the central circulation (the heart and the pulmonary circulation), and (2) the systemic circulation (loosely defined as all vascular beds fed from the aorta). This is to our advantage because it is helpful to study the two major subdivisions of the system separately and then to put our knowledge together for a complete picture of the cardiovascular system. The heart, of course, functions as the body's vascular pump, transferring blood from the low-pressure systemic veins to the high-pressure systemic arteries. In this process, the heart pumps the blood through the pulmonary circulation where gas exchange occurs.

Although the heart is usually described in singular terms there are actually two separate hearts, the left and the right, although they are in intimate proximity to each other, sharing a common wall. The right heart, interposed between the systemic veins and the pulmonary artery, pumps blood from the systemic circulation into the pulmonary circulation. Except for minor beat-to-beat variations, the blood pumped by each heart per minute must be equal, as can be expected from a closed-circuit

31

system. Indeed, at any given time the flow at each and every point in the circulation must be equal. This is an inevitable consequence of a closed system.* It is because the left and right hearts pump the same quantity of blood under steady-state conditions that we can conceptually lump the two hearts and the pulmonary circulation together into a single unit usually referred to as the central circulation.

The two principal mechanical properties of the circulatory system that must be considered in any conceptual schema are compliance and resistance, i.e. the volume-pressure and pressure-flow relationships. All vessels have both compliance and resistance. However, each function is not equally important at each serial segment of the circulation. This is because of anatomic differences as we go from aorta to vena cava (or from pulmonary artery to pulmonary vein). These anatomic differences have profound functional significance.

Table 2 summarizes the basic properties of the various serial sections of the systemic circulation.[6] The aorta and large distributing arteries possess a great deal of elastic tissue. Because of this their elastance is high; therefore their compliance is low (Chap. 1). The function of the aorta is principally conductance; that of the distributing arteries is resistance. The arterioles also possess elastic tissue, although less than the aorta and distributing arteries. What the arterioles may lack in elastic tissue they more than make up with a thick coat of vascular smooth muscle. When contracted this smooth muscle produces what is generally referred to as vascular or arteriolar tone. The arterioles have low compliance. Their function is principally resistance; however, many physiologists have suggested the arterioles also produce the effective back pressure for the arterial system (Chap. 6). The smallest venules possess no elastic tissue. However, small amounts of elastic tissue begin to reappear in the larger venules and small veins. As a group, the small veins and venules have little elastance and a large compliance. Toward the downstream end of the systemic circulation in the large veins and vena cava, elastic tissue is found in large amounts. The compliance of this segment of the venous system is less than that of the small veins and venules and its function is resistance. Thus, only one serial section of the systemic circulation (the small veins and venules) has significant compliance. Because the veins (principally the

---

*Although the flow at each point in the circulation at any given point in time must remain constant, the velocity (v) must vary at each point in the system depending upon the cross-sectional area (A), i.e. $v = \dot{Q}/A$.

Table 2. Summary of the Basic Properties of the Various Serial Sections of the Systemic Circulation

Vessel	Mean Pressure (mm Hg)	Amount of Elastic Tissue	Primary Function
Aorta	90–110	+ + + +	Conductive
Distributing arteries	80–90	+ + + +	Resistive
Arterioles	40–60	+ +	Resistive (effective back pressure)
		(mostly smooth muscle)	
Capillary	15–25	0	Exchange
Small veins and venules	5–10	0– +	Capacitive
		(reappears in large venules)	
Large veins and vena cava	0–2	+ + +	Resistive

small veins and venules) have the capacity to hold large volumes of blood (Chap. 3), they are called the capacitance vessels. The arterial vessels on the other hand are called conductance (e.g. the aorta) or resistance (e.g. small arteries and arterioles) vessels, depending upon their size.

Although the primary function of the venous system is capacitive, the resistance to flow within the large veins is nevertheless most significant. The function of the venous resistance is entirely different from that of the arterial resistance. Whereas the arteriolar tone serves to maintain an elevated arterial blood pressure and to distribute flow between parallel channels, the venous resistance serves as a major determinant of the amount of blood returning to the heart. This venous function is so important that it will be discussed in greater detail in the next chapter.

The reasons for conceptually placing the venous resistance downstream from the major systemic capacitance area are based not only upon the relatively low compliance of this venous segment (large veins and vena cava) but also upon functional evidence.[8,3] If the arterial flow into the systemic circulation was suddenly stopped (e.g. by clamping the aorta), blood entering the right atrium would not stop instantly but would continue to flow, the rate decreasing in an exponential manner, for several minutes. This behavior can be accounted for only by a significant resistance to flow between the capacitance area (the vascular reservoir) and the right atrium.

Although the resistance and compliance values of the pulmonary circulation are quantitatively different from those of the systemic circulation,* evidence suggests that the same basic conceptual schema can be applied (Chap. 7). Thus, the pulmonary arteries and large pulmonary veins are considered primarily resistance vessels whereas the small pulmonary veins and venules are considered the capacitance vessels.

In developing this conceptual schema of the circulation the capillary segment of the systemic circulation has been ignored. This is because its primary function is that of exchange, the capillaries having little effect on the overall hemodynamics of the circulation except insofar as volume can leave or enter the circulation through the capillaries.

Presented in Figure 12 is a schematic drawing of the circulatory system known as a lumped parameter model. It is based on the mechanical properties of the circulatory system discussed above. The term *lumped parameter* indicates that all the many parallel vascular beds have been conceptually lumped together into a single equivalent channel. This circulatory system has been further lumped together into its two major subdivisions: the systemic circulation and the central circulation (composed of the two hearts and the pulmonary circulation). Each serial segment is considered to have only its primary hemodynamic function. Thus, the arterial system and large veins and vena cava are depicted as tubes whereas the small veins and venules are depicted as a compliant sac. The corresponding segments of the pulmonary system are depicted similarly. As this conceptual model is designed to illustrate the important hemodynamic characteristics of the circulatory system, the capillary beds have been excluded. A comparable hydraulic model of the circulatory system is presented in Figure 13.

----

*Representative values of the pulmonary and systemic resistance and compliances determined in the dog are as follows. Systemic arterial resistance = 58.1 mm $Hg \cdot l^{-1} \cdot min$; pulmonary arterial resistance = 9.4 mm $Hg \cdot l^{-1}$ min; lumped systemic compliance = 2.6 ml $\cdot kg^{-1} \cdot mm$ Hg^{-1}; lumped pulmonary compliance = 0.1 ml $\cdot kg^{-1} \cdot mm$ Hg; systemic venous resistance = 4.4 mm $Hg \cdot l^{-1} \cdot min$; and pulmonary venous resistance = 0.6 mm $Hg \cdot l^{-1} \cdot min$.

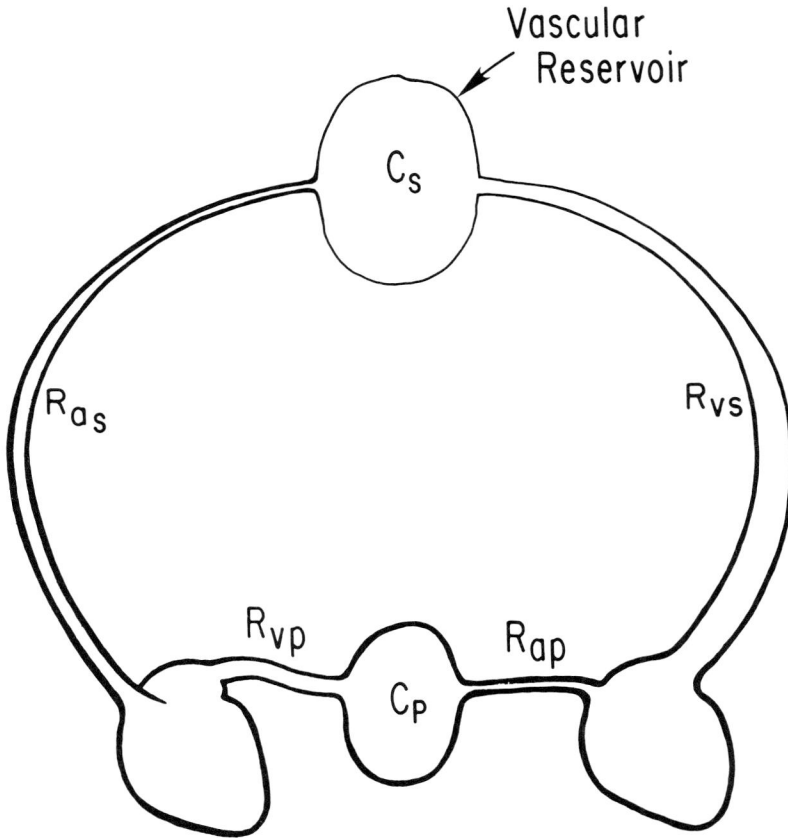

Fig. 12. Lumped parameter model of the circulatory system. R_{AS} = systemic arterial resistance, R_{AP} = pulmonary arterial resistance, R_{VS} = systemic venous resistance, R_{VP} = pulmonary venous resistance, C_S = systemic vascular compliance, and C_P = pulmonary vascular compliance.

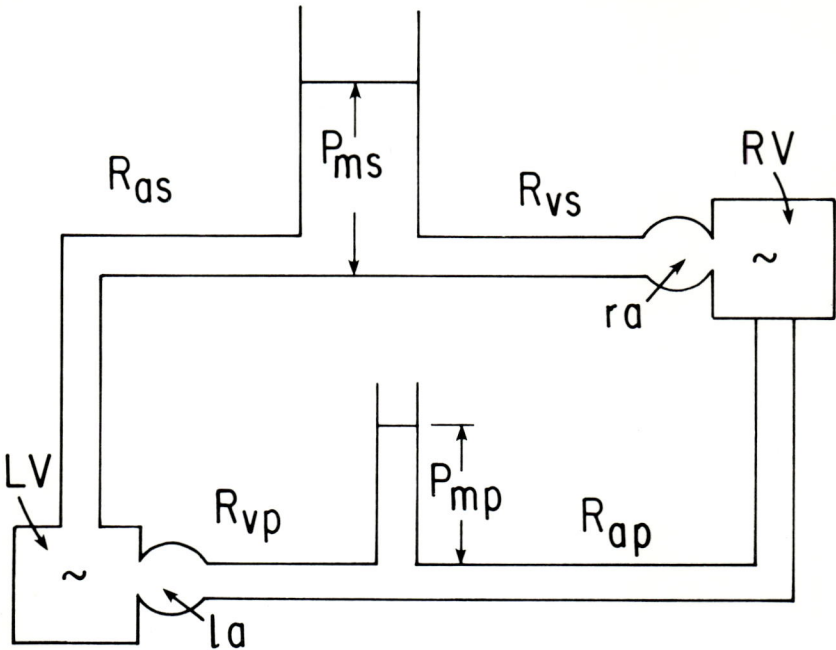

Fig. 13.   Hydraulic model of the circulatory system. R_{AS} = systemic arterial resistance, R_{AP} = pulmonary arterial resistance, R_{VS} = systemic venous resistance, R_{VP} = pulmonary venous resistance, P_{MS} = mean systemic pressure, P_{MP} = mean pulmonary pressure, ra = right atrium, RV = right ventricle, la = left atrium, and LV = left ventricle.

Although these models may seem unrealistic, that is, they lump all the many parallel channels together and exclude the capillaries, they nevertheless possess many of the significant characteristics of the cardiovascular system, as shown in the next chapter. They, thus, provide a useful conceptual framework upon which to hang modifying bits and pieces of information.

To summarize, both systemic arteries and veins have resistive and capacitive functions; the relative magnitudes of these functions depend principally upon structural differences. The function of resistance may be found within the arterial system and at the outflow of the venous system. The function of capacitance is dominant at the level of the small veins and venules. The next chapter will deal with the hemodynamic consequences arising from the structure of the systemic circulation.

5

Pressure-flow Relationships of the Systemic Venous System

THE VASCULAR RESERVOIR

To begin our description of the pressure-flow relationships of the systemic venous system, it is appropriate to discuss the importance of the reservoir function of the veins. In order for any pump to operate, there must be some fluid to pump! This, of course, is of fundamental significance. Consider the example illustrated in Figure 14. If one were to take a simple hand pump, such as a sailboat bilge pump which operates on the stroke-volume principle,* and attach the same single rigid tube to both the inflow and outflow ends of the pump (Fig. 14) he would be unable to pump any fluid because there would be no fluid for the pump to take up; the system is rigid. If, however, the rigid tube were cut in half and a reservoir interposed between the cut ends from which the pump could obtain fluid, not only would the pump be operable but also the amount of fluid that could be pumped would be limited only by the number of strokes per minute. The heart is not really any different from the bilge pump. It needs a reservoir of blood from which it can draw the blood to be pumped. Fortunately, the highly compliant veins (the small veins and venules) provide this necessary *vascular reservoir*.

---

*Fluid is taken up into the pumping chamber during a period of relaxation, then ejected during a period of activation.

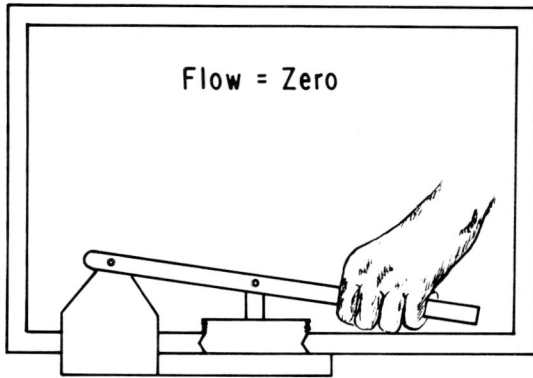

(a)

Flow = Zero

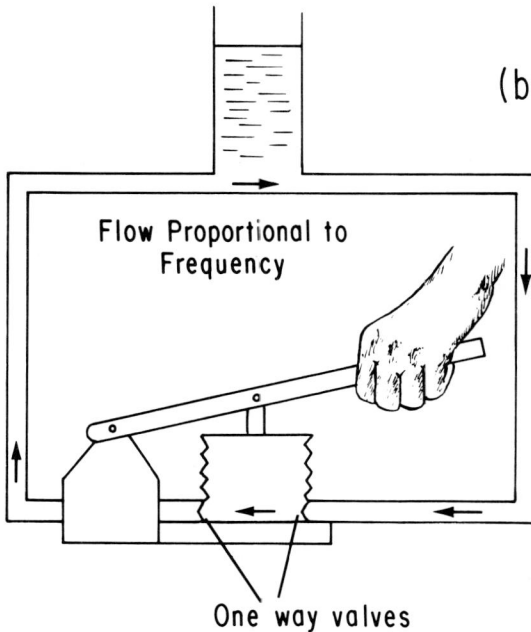

(b)

Flow Proportional to
Frequency

One way valves

Fig. 14. Schematic illustrating the mechanism of operation of a stroke-volume pump. *a:* When the pump is connected in series with a rigid system there is no fluid available to prime the pump; therefore flow is zero. *b:* When the pump is connected in series with a reservoir, fluid may be taken into the pumping chamber from the reservoir during the relaxation phase of the pumping cycle and ejected into the reservoir during the active phase of the cycle. In general the greater the frequency of the pumping cycle the greater will be the flow, until the frequency becomes high enough to limit the period of inflow to such an extent that the chamber is not filled completely during the relaxation phase.

DETERMINANTS OF VENOUS RETURN

As discussed in Chapter 2, before there can be any flow there must be a pressure gradient, i.e. an upstream pressure minus a downstream pressure. The upstream driving pressure for venous return is the pressure at the inflow to the venous system, the pressure within the small veins and venules which is equal to the static mean systemic pressure, P_{MS} (Chap. 3). To say it another way, under static conditions (when venous return equals zero) the downstream (right atrial) pressure rises to equal the upstream driving pressure (the mean systemic pressure, i.e. the pressure within the small veins and venules) for venous return. The mean systemic pressure is determined by the blood volume and the elastic properties of the systemic circulation (Chaps. 3 and 4) and is defined as follows:*

$$P_{MS} = \frac{V - V_0}{C_S},\qquad(10)$$

where C_S = systemic vascular compliance, mostly that of the small veins and venules (ml/mm Hg); V_0 = unstressed vascular volume (ml), which is the volume contained in the vascular reservoir when the mean systemic pressure is atmospheric; and V = the total vascular volume (ml). $V-V_0$ is thus the stressed volume of the circulatory system (volume above V_0).

The downstream pressure for venous return is the pressure at the outflow to the venous system. Under conditions where right atrial pressure, P_{RA}, is greater than atmospheric pressure, P_{ATM}, right atrial pressure is the effective downstream pressure. (For convenience, the atmospheric pressure is always considered to be zero.) When right atrial pressure falls to a subatmospheric value, the great veins entering the chest collapse at their point of entry into the chest, isolating the right atrium from the rest of the splanchnic circulation. Under these conditions, the great veins, at their point of entry into the chest, function as Starling resistors, i.e. their internal pressure becomes fixed at the effective surrounding pressure which is atmospheric pressure (Chap. 2). Atmospheric pressure, therefore, becomes the effective downstream pressure whenever the right atrial pressure falls to subatmospheric values.

---

*Compare this expression with Equation 3, Chapter 1.

Knowing the driving pressures we can write an expression describing the pressure-flow relationship of the venous system as follows:

Whenever

$$P_{RA} > P_{ATM}$$

$$\dot{Q} = \frac{P_{MS} - P_{RA}}{R_{VS}} \qquad (11)$$

and whenever

$$P_{RA} \leq P_{ATM}$$

$$\dot{Q} = \frac{P_{MS} - P_{ATM}}{R_{VS}} . \qquad (12)$$

In these equations, $\dot{Q}$ = venous return (l/min); R_{VS} = systemic venous resistance, i.e. the resistance to flow of the large veins and vena cava (mm Hg·l^{-1}·min); and P_{MS}, P_{RA}, and P_{ATM} (mm Hg) are defined as above. Graphic solutions to Equations 11 and 12 are presented in Figure 15 for both positive (Eq. 11) and negative (Eq. 12) values of right atrial pressure. The resulting curve, known as the *venous return curve*, represents all possible combinations of venous return and right atrial pressure. If one understands the shape and position of the venous return curve one understands the determinants of venous return.

Since volume and the elastic characteristics of the systemic circulation are the determinants of the mean systemic pressure, any consideration of the determinants of venous return must also entail the consideration of the volume-pressure relationship of the systemic circulation. Thus, an increase in V would increase P_{MS} and, therefore, venous return. A decrease in V_0 and C_S would

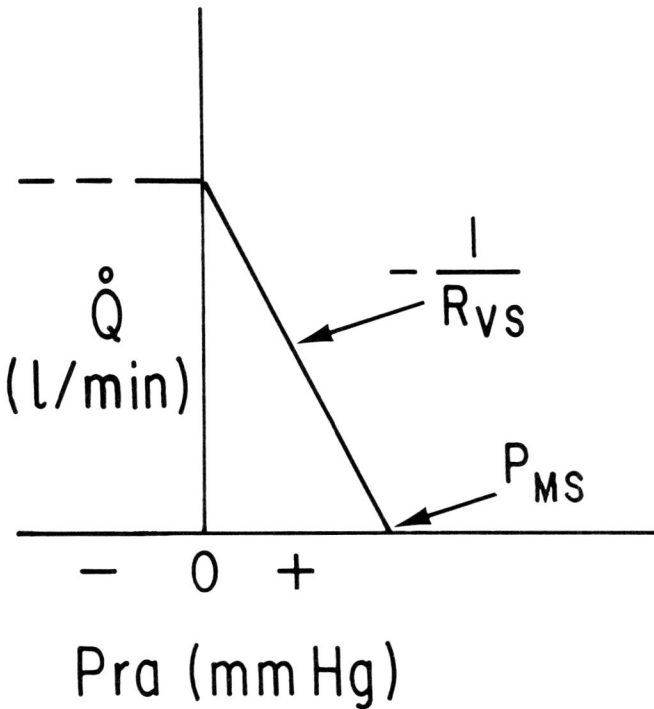

Fig. 15. Graphic solutions to Equation 11 (solid line) and Equation 12 (dashed line). Right atrial pressure (P_{RA}) is plotted on the abscissa and venous return ($\dot{Q}$) on the ordinate. The resulting curve known as the *venous return curve* describes the pressure-flow relationships of the venous system. The slope of the venous return curve is equal to minus the reciprocal of the systemic venous resistance (R_{VS}). When $\dot{Q}$ is equal to zero, P_{RA} (the downstream pressure) rises to equal P_{MS} (the upstream driving pressure for venous return). As P_{RA} is lowered the pressure gradient for venous return ($P_{MS} - P_{RA}$) increases and so does venous return. When P_{RA} falls below zero (the dashed line) the great veins entering the chest collapse at their point of entry into the chest. At this point the pressure within the veins becomes fixed at atmospheric pressure (0), and the pressure gradient for venous return becomes fixed at its maximal value. Venous return, therefore, does not increase even when P_{RA} is lowered to a negative (subatmospheric) value. For venous return to increase further when $P_{RA} \leq 0$, either P_{MS} must increase (Fig. 16) or R_V must decrease (Fig. 17).

also increase P_{MS} and venous return. An increase in V can be accomplished simply by a transfusion. A decrease in V_O or C_S requires a contraction of the vascular smooth muscle located within the walls of the small veins and venules. This can be accomplished either by vasoconstrictor agents circulating in the blood or by direct action of the sympathetic nerves. The effects that changes in the mean systemic pressure have on the venous return curve are illustrated in Figure 16.

The systemic venous resistance (R_{VS}) also has a profound effect upon venous return. An increase in this resistance would decrease venous return while a decrease would increase venous

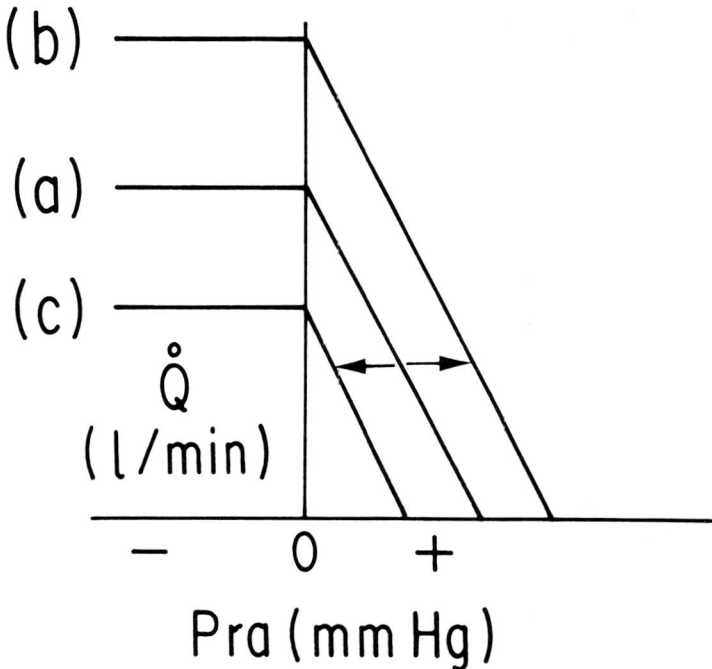

Fig. 16.   This figure illustrates the effects that changes in mean systemic pressure, P_{MS} (P_{RA} at zero $\dot{Q}$), can have on the venous return curve. Increasing P_{MS} (curve *b*) shifts the venous return curve to the right increasing venous return ($\dot{Q}$) at any level of P_{RA}. Decreasing P_{MS} (curve *c*) shifts the venous return curve to the left, decreasing $\dot{Q}$ at any level of P_{RA}. An increase in P_{MS} can be brought about by an increase in the stressed vascular volume, a decrease in the unstressed vascular volume, or a decrease in systemic compliance (Eq. 10). Similarly, opposite changes in these parameters will decrease P_{MS} and, therefore, $\dot{Q}$.

return. An increase in the systemic venous resistance can be achieved either by a contraction of the smooth muscles within the walls of the large veins or by external compression, such as may occur with an abdominal tumor or a pregnancy. The effects that changes in the systemic venous resistance have on the venous return curve are illustrated in Figure 17.

Thus, contraction of the systemic veins can have opposite effects on venous return; depending upon whether the small

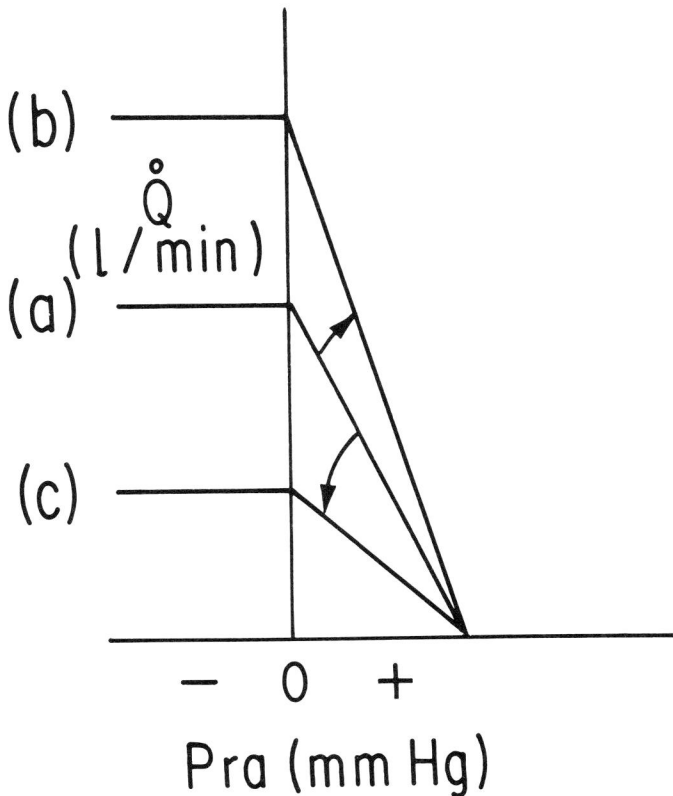

Fig. 17.   This figure illustrates the effects that changes in systemic venous resistance (R_{VS}) have on the venous return curve. Increasing R_{VS} (curve c) decreases the slope of the venous return curve, decreasing venous return ($\dot{Q}$) at any level of right atrial pressure (P_{RA}). Decreasing R_{VS} (curve b) increases the slope of the venous return curve, increasing $\dot{Q}$ at any level of P_{RA}. An increase in R_{VS} can be achieved by a contraction of vascular smooth muscles within the walls of the large veins or from external compression. A decrease in R_{VS} will occur with an elevated blood volume which increases transmural pressure of the veins, thus increasing their radius.

veins and venules or the larger veins contracted. A contraction of the small veins and venules will decrease V_0 and C_S, increasing $\dot{Q}$. A contraction of the large veins will increase R_{VS} and decrease $\dot{Q}$.

EFFECT OF GRAVITY ON VENOUS RETURN

The systemic venous return was described by Equation 11 as the ratio of the difference between the mean systemic and right atrial pressures divided by the venous resistance, where the mean systemic pressure is assumed to be the transmural pressure of the systemic vascular reservoir. The implicit assumption of Equation 11 is that all areas of the circulation are in the horizontal plane. Since the vascular reservoir is predominantly composed of those areas inferior to the heart (i.e. the splanchnic area, all vascular areas which drain through the liver), the upstream driving pressure for venous return (the mean systemic pressure) must be modified by the hydrostatic factor ρgh (Chap. 2) whenever the circulation is rotated above or below the level of the right atrium (the outflow of the systemic circulation) or whenever the systemic circulation is subjected to an acceleration stress in the same plane as the circulation. Here ρ is the density of blood, g is the magnitude of the gravitation or acceleration stress, h is the distance separating the vascular reservoir from the heart. When the circulation is tilted above or below the horizontal plane an effective mean systemic pressure, $P_{MS\ eff}$, replaces P_{MS} in Equations 11 and 12, where

$$P_{MS\ eff} = P_{MS} \pm \rho gh. \tag{13}$$

When the feet are at a higher horizontal level than the heart, or with negative acceleration (i.e. acceleration stress in the direction of the head), $P_{MS\ eff} = P_{MS} + \rho gh$; when the feet are at a lower horizontal level than the heart, or with positive acceleration (i.e. acceleration stress in the direction of the feet), $P_{MS\ eff} = P_{MS} - \rho gh$. Substituting Equation 13 into Equation 11,

$$\dot{Q} = \frac{(P_{MS} \pm \rho gh) - P_{RA}}{R_{VS}}, \tag{14}$$

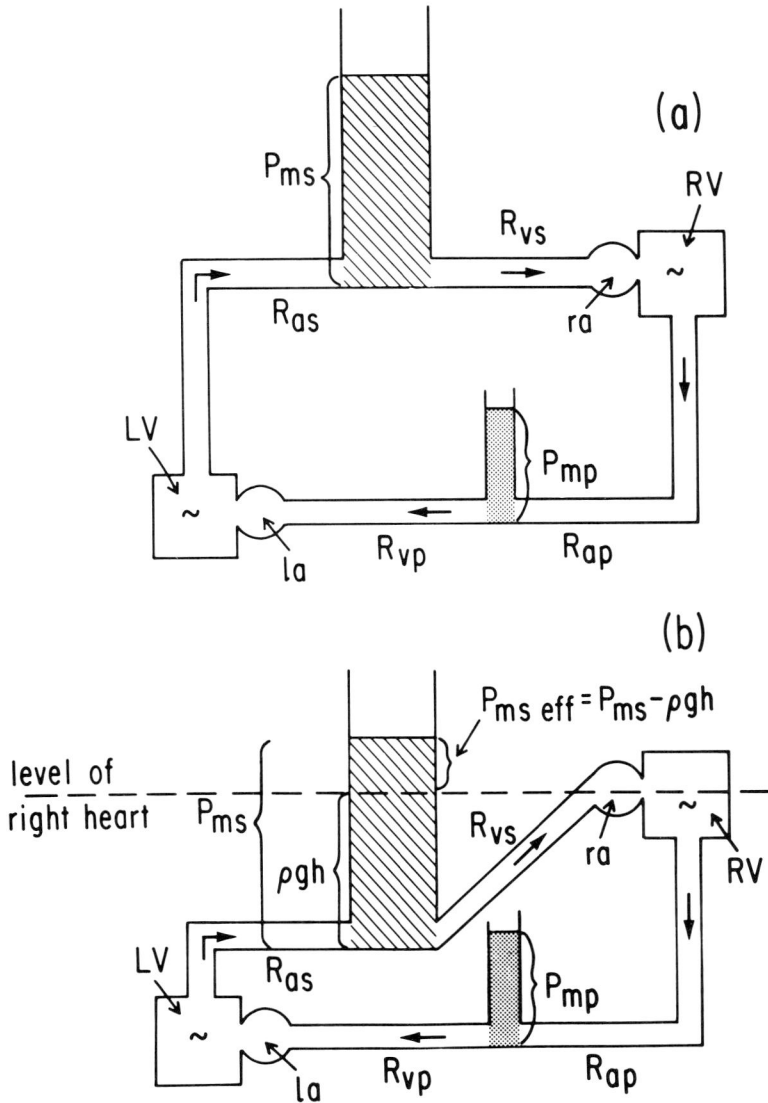

Fig. 18. Hydraulic model of the circulatory system illustrates the effect of tilting (acceleration stress) on the systemic circulation. Imagine this figure as three dimensional with both the right and left hearts on the same horizontal plane. *a:* The normal condition when all parts of the circulatory system are in the same plane (no acceleration stress). *b:* A feet-down tilt (positive acceleration stress) when much of the systemic blood volume (ρgh) falls (is pooled) below heart level. During a feet-down tilt the effective pressure driving blood back to the heart, P_{MSeff}, is $P_{MS} - \rho gh$. RV = right ventricle, LV = left ventricle, ra = right atrium, la = left atrium, R_{AP} and R_{AS} = arterial resistances of the pulmonary and systemic circuits, respectively, R_{VP} and R_{VS} = venous resistances of the pulmonary and systemic circuits, respectively, while P_{MP} and P_{MS} are the mean pulmonary and mean systemic pressures.

which describes the pressure-flow relationships of the systemic venous system under the influence of gravity. Since the lungs essentially surround the heart, gravity does not affect the total pulmonary venous return to the extent that it affects the systemic venous return. Gravity, however, does significantly affect the pressure-flow relationships of the individual pulmonary capillaries, as will be discussed in Chapter 7.

Figure 18 illustrates the effect of gravity on the systemic circulation using the hydraulic model presented in Figure 13. In this figure, when the vascular reservoir is lowered below the level of the heart (i.e. when a human rotates from supine to standing position), the effective upstream driving pressure for venous return is reduced by an amount proportional to the degree of rotation. The amount of volume in the reservoir which is rotated below heart level is generally referred to as the "pooled" volume. It is essentially a volume which produces a pressure (ρgh) which does not partake in the generation of a pressure gradient for flow. If it were not for compensating factors, venous return in the human would abruptly drop toward zero when the vertical position is assumed. This is because most of the volume in the vascular reservoir (mostly inferior to the heart) would fall (be "pooled") below the heart level. Various reflexes, however, come into play to return the effective mean systemic pressure back toward normal. These mechanisms will be discussed in Chapter 9.

In summary, venous return is a function of the stressed volume of the systemic circulation and the elastic-resistive characteristics of the venous system. To say it another way, the elastic recoil of the small veins and venules produces the mean systemic pressure which propels blood back to the heart against the resistance of the large veins and vena cava. When the circulatory system is rotated in a gravitational field or subject to an acceleration stress, the mean systemic pressure is either increased or decreased depending upon the direction of rotation or of acceleration.

6

Pressure-flow Relationships of the Arterial System

In the preceding chapters we learned how the pressure gradient for venous return is a function of the elastic properties of the vascular reservoir (small veins and venules) and the blood volume of the reservoir. We also discussed how venous return must be equal to cardiac output since the circulatory system is a closed circuit. The arterial system completes the circuit by returning to the vascular reservoir the blood volume which is pumped by the heart. The arterial system also has another important function—that of distributing the cardiac output to the various parallel channels in proportion to their metabolic needs. Thus, exercising skeletal muscles may receive more blood flow than a quiescent intestine. This is accomplished by active alterations in the pressure-flow relationships of the arterial system.*

ARTERIAL PRESSURE-FLOW RELATIONSHIPS

The pressure-flow relationships of the arterial system can be described by an application of the Poiseuille equation (Eq. 5),

$$\dot{Q} = \frac{1}{R}(P_I - P_O) .$$ (5)

---

*Recall from our earlier discussion (Chaps. 3 and 4) that systemic arterial compliance is about 0.07 ml·kg^{-1}·mm Hg^{-1}, whereas systemic venous compliance is about 2.6 ml·kg^{-1}·mm Hg^{-1}. Therefore, the arterial system has principally a resistive function.

47

The inflow pressure (P_I) is the arterial pressure (P_a). The outflow pressure (P_O) depends upon the exact conceptual model of the arterial system one chooses. For the lumped parameter model discussed in Chapter 5, the arterial pressure-flow relationships may be described by the following application of Poiseuille's equation:

$$\dot{Q} = \frac{1}{R_a} (P_a - P_{MS}) \, , \tag{15}$$

where $\dot{Q}$ = cardiac output, P_a = arterial (aortic) pressure, P_{MS} = mean system pressure (the pressure in the vascular reservoir), and R_a = the arterial resistance (the resistance to flow between the aorta and the small veins and venules). Many physiologists write but one flow equation for the entire systemic circulation, i.e.

$$\dot{Q} = \frac{1}{TPR} (P_a - P_{RA}) \, , \tag{16}$$

where $\dot{Q}$ = cardiac output, P_a = arterial pressure, P_{RA} = right atrial pressure, and TPR = total peripheral resistance, the resistance across the entire peripheral circulation from aorta to right atrium. Both Equations 15 and 16 have been used to describe arterial pressure-flow relationships. Since the largest pressure drop across the circulatory system occurs with the arteries and arterioles, Equation 16 largely reflects this pressure drop. However, unlike Equation 15, this latter expression also reflects changes in venous resistance, and for this reason many physiologists in recent years have preferred Equation 15.

Although we tend to think of arterial resistance in terms of the lumped parameter model, i.e. as a single resistance channel, the resistance calculated from the above equation actually represents an average resistance of the many parallel vascular channels. We can, however, study the arterial resistance characteristics of the individual organs of the body by isolating and perfusing those organs separately. When this is done three major types of arterial pressure-flow relationships become evident, which are depicted in Figure 19.

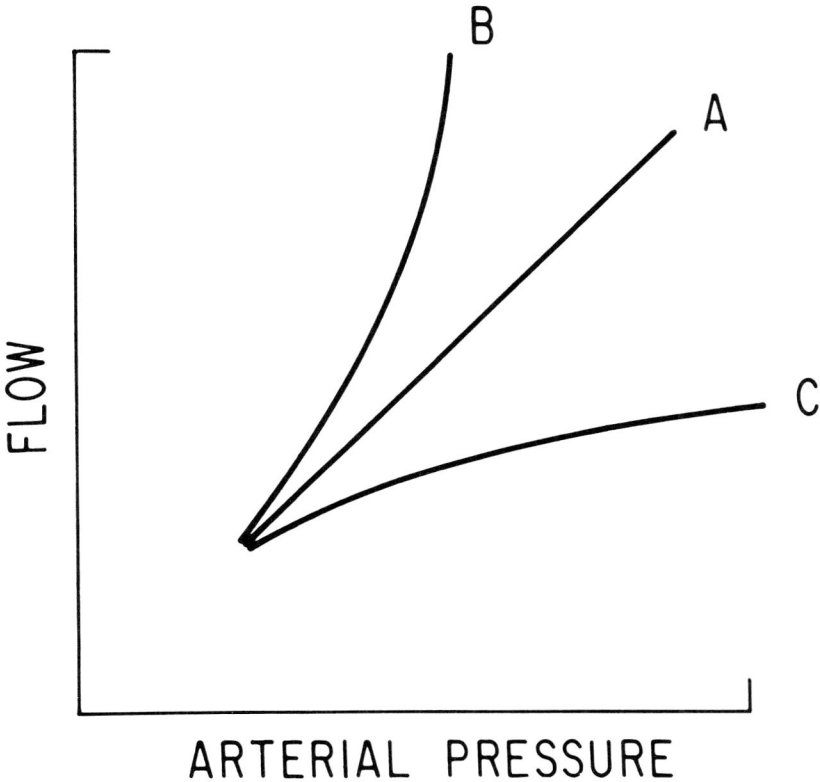

Fig. 19. The three major types of arterial pressure-flow relationships. Curve A depicts an arterial bed that functions as a rigid tube. Curve B depicts an arterial bed that responds passively to an increasing arterial pressure by dilating. Curve C depicts an arterial bed that responds actively to an increasing arterial pressure by constricting. The latter response is referred to as autoregulation.

The slope of these curves is equal to the reciprocal of the arterial resistance. Therefore, an increase in arterial resistance decreases the slope of the arterial pressure-flow relationship, whereas a decrease in arterial resistance increases the slope. Curve A (Fig. 19) represents an arterial system that would function as a rigid tube, i.e. changes in arterial transmural pressure have no effect on arterial resistance. This linear relationship is not common in the arterial system. Curve B (Fig. 19) represents a vascular bed which responds passively to an increase in arterial distending pressure by arterial dilation, which reduces the arterial resistance. The greater the arterial pressure, the less the resistance. Curve C (Fig. 19) represents a vascular bed which responds actively to an increase in distending pressure by constricting the arteries, increasing the resistance to flow. This latter type of response is so common and so important that it has been given the name of *autoregulation*. It is the homeostatic* process by which a vascular bed maintains its blood flow relatively constant despite changes in perfusion pressure. Autoregulation of blood flow occurs in such essential organs as the brain, kidney, heart, skeletal muscles and intestine.

CONCEPT OF THE EFFECTIVE BACK PRESSURE

As stated previously, several back pressures have been used in the Poiseuille equation (Eq. 5), depending upon the exact conceptual model chosen. Either the mean systemic pressure or the right atrial pressure has been the back pressure used by most physiologists. The use of these back pressures implies that the circulatory system, particularly the arterial system, functions as a rigid tube. As this is clearly not the case, Permutt and Riley[28] recently extended the principles of the Starling resistor to arterioles by suggesting that active tension in the smooth muscles in the walls of arterioles functioned as an inward-acting pressure, analogous to the pressure surrounding a collapsible tube. In their model, under conditions where $\dot{Q} = 0$, this inward-acting pressure manifests itself as a critical closing pressure† as suggested by Burton,[7] much as P_1 equals P_s in the Starling resistor when $\dot{Q} = 0$ (Eq. 6). Under conditions of flow, when the capillary pressure (P_O) is less then the critical closing pressure, this inward-acting pressure manifests itself as the "effective" back pressure to perfusion, P_C', much as the surrounding pressure does in a Starling resistor when the outflow pressure is less than the surrounding pressure. The pressure-flow relationships through the arterial system can, therefore, be

---

Homeostasis is the word coined by Cannon[9] to describe the process by which the body maintains an almost unvarying cellular environment, *le milieu interieur* described earlier by Claude Bernard.[5]

†Burton defined the critical closing pressure of a vascular bed as the arterial pressure when $\dot{Q} = 0$. Critical closing pressure can be measured in isolated vascular beds by occluding arterial inflow and measuring arterial pressure distal to the occlusion. Arterial pressure after flow is occluded rapidly falls to a plateau value greater than venous pressure. Critical closing pressures as high as 30 to 40 mm Hg are not unusual.

described by Equation 15 by allowing P_C' to replace P_S as the back-pressure. Thus:

$$\dot{Q} = \frac{P_a - P'_C}{R_a} . \qquad (17)$$

The resistance to flow in this case would depend upon the dimensions of the vessel up to, but not including, the area of critical closure.*

Burton[7] defined the critical closing pressure (P_C') by an application of the law of La Place as follows:

$$P'_C = \frac{T_A}{r_0} , \qquad (18)$$

where T_A = active tension (vascular smooth muscle tone), r_0 = unstretched radius.† Substituting Equation 18 into Equation 17 yields:

$$\dot{Q} = \frac{1}{R_a} P_a - \frac{T_A}{r_0}. \qquad (19)$$

This equation allows one to predict the pressure-flow relationships that a vascular bed with tone would have if it behaved in a manner analogous to a Starling resistor with the active tone acting as an equivalent surrounding pressure, i.e. the effective back pressure. To illustrate this, Equation 19 was solved graphically in Figure 20A for the relationship between P_a and $\dot{Q}$ at constant T_A and r_0. R_a and r_0 were held constant at one, while T_A was assigned the values of 10, 20, and 30. P_0 was assumed to remain at atmospheric pressure. When $\dot{Q} = 0$, $P_a = P_C'$. Note that

---

*Since various resistances have been used to describe arterial pressure-flow relationships confusion as to which one is meant may result. If this occurs simply remember that a resistance is defined by a pressure drop divided by a flow. Establish which pressure drop is used and you will have defined the resistance.

†Units of T_A/r_0 are dynes/cm² which is a pressure.

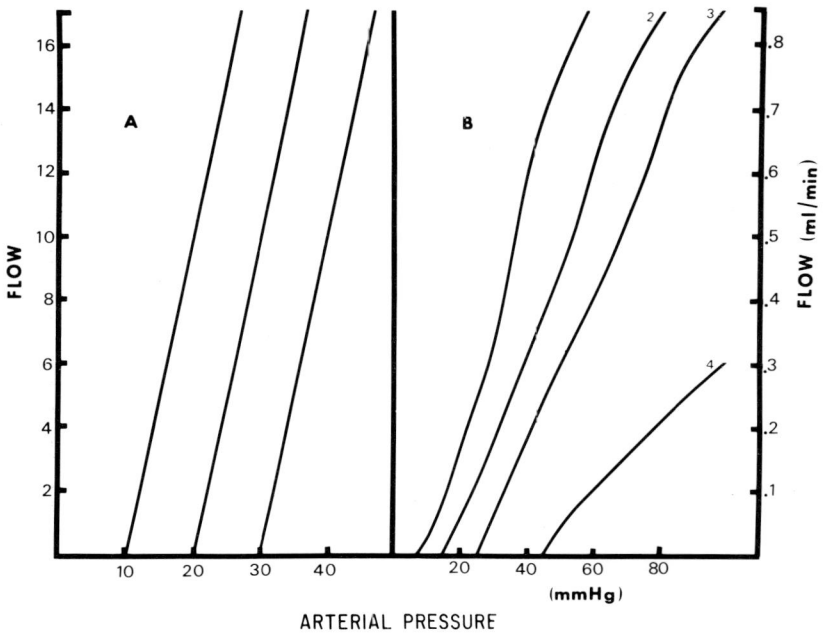

Fig. 20. Comparison of experimentally obtained pressure-flow curves to the pressure-flow relationships theoretically expected if a vascular bed behaved analogously to a Starling resistor, with the active tone acting as an equivalent surrounding pressure. In A theoretically derived curves are drawn and in B actual data curves obtained from the rabbit's hind limb by Nichol et al. (Fundamental instability of small blood vessels and central closing pressures in vascular beds. Am. J. Physiol., *164*:330, 1951) are replotted. The abscissa is the arterial pressure.

no flow occurs until $P_a > P_C'$; thereafter flow increases linearly with P_a. The effect of increasing active tone (T_A) is to shift the pressure-flow curve to the right without affecting the slope, which is the reciprocal of the resistance, i.e. increasing the effective back pressure. Figure 20B, replotted from Nichol et al. (1951) serves as an example of the pressure-flow relationships of a typical vascular bed under conditions of increasing vascular tone. These data were obtained from the rabbit's hind limb when the venous pressure was zero. Curves 1 to 4 represent increasing vasomotor tone produced by electrical stimulation of sympathetic nerves at increasing frequencies. Notice that increasing the vasomotor tone leads to a shifting of the pressure-flow curves to the right with only a slight change in slopes until very high degrees of tone are produced, i.e. increasing the vasomotor tone leads to an increase in the effective back pressure.

In summary, the arterial system seldom functions as a rigid system. Increasing the arterial pressure passively distends the arteries, decreasing arterial resistance. Conversely, decreasing the arterial pressure passively increases the arterial resistance. Arteriolar tone causes arteries to function in a manner analogous to Starling resistors by generating an effective arterial back pressure greater than capillary pressure. By adjusting arterial resistance (and/or the effective arterial back pressure), the circulatory system can distribute cardiac output to the organs where the flow is most needed.

7

Pressure-flow Relationships of the Pulmonary Circulation

THE STARLING RESISTOR CONCEPT APPLIED TO THE PULMONARY CIRCULATION

The important feature of the pulmonary circulation is the collapsible nature of the pulmonary capillaries. Thin walled and surrounded by alveolar pressure, these capillaries are able to function as Starling resistors. In fact, the pulmonary circulation is the classical example of the physiologic importance of collapsible tubes (Chap. 2).

In Chapter 2 we summarized the pressure-flow relationships through an ideal Starling resistor by the following three succinct statements: (1) Whenever the pressure surrounding a collapsible tube is greater than the inflow pressure which, in turn, is greater than the outflow pressure, no flow occurs through the tube. (2) Whenever surrounding pressure is greater than outflow pressure, flow is proportional to the difference between inflow pressure and surrounding pressure, and changes in outflow pressure have no influence on flow. (3) Whenever outflow pressure is greater than surrounding pressure, flow is proportional to the difference between inflow pressure and outflow pressure, and changes in surrounding pressure have no influence on flow. The three possible conditions of a Starling resistor were depicted as hydraulic models in Figure 7.

Since the pulmonary capillaries are collapsible tubes, the pressure-flow relationships through pulmonary capillaries may be described by the above three statements if the following substitutions are made: pulmonary arterial pressure for inflow pressure, pulmonary venous pressure for outflow pressure, and alveolar pressure for surrounding pressure. Thus: (1) Whenever the alveolar pressure surrounding a pulmonary capillary is greater than the pulmonary artery pressure which, in turn, is greater than the pulmonary venous pressure, no flow occurs through the capillary. (2) Whenever alveolar pressure is greater than pulmonary venous pressure, but is less than pulmonary arterial pressure, flow is proportional to the difference between pulmonary arterial pressure and alveolar pressure, and changes in pulmonary venous pressure have no influence on flow. (3) Whenever pulmonary venous pressure is greater than alveolar pressure, flow is proportional to the difference between pulmonary arterial pressure and pulmonary venous pressure, and changes in alveolar pressure have no influence on flow.

Studies demonstrating that the pressure-flow relationships of the pulmonary circulation are analogous to those of a Starling resistor were done originally in dog lungs.[27,39,40] Figure 21 presents the pressure-flow relationships obtained by Permutt, Bromberger, and Bane.[27] They cannulated the pulmonary veins of the left lower lobe of a lung in an anesthetized dog with the chest open, and recorded changes in flow as the venous pressure was very slowly changed. Plotted on the ordinate is venous return from the lobe, and on the abscissa pulmonary venous pressure. Three curves are shown. The left-hand curve was obtained at an alveolar pressure of 3 mm Hg and a pulmonary artery pressure of 19 mm Hg. The middle curve was obtained at an alveolar pressure of 10 mm Hg and a pulmonary artery pressure of 29 mm Hg. The right-hand curve was obtained at an alveolar pressure of 18 mm Hg and a pulmonary artery pressure of 38 mm Hg. In general, flow increased as outflow pressure (pulmonary venous pressure) was lowered at constant inflow pressure (pulmonary arterial pressure) until outflow pressure was lower below the pressure surrounding the pulmonary capillaries (alveolar pressure). As outflow pressure was lowered further, flow decreased slightly although this is not the significant feature of these curves. These curves all have the same general shape as that presented in Figure 8C, which considered a theoretical Starling resistor. They are also similar to a systemic venous return curve in which the inflection can be accounted for in terms of veins collapsing as they enter the chest.

Evidence that the Starling resistor concept can be used to interpret the pressure-flow relationships of the pulmonary circu-

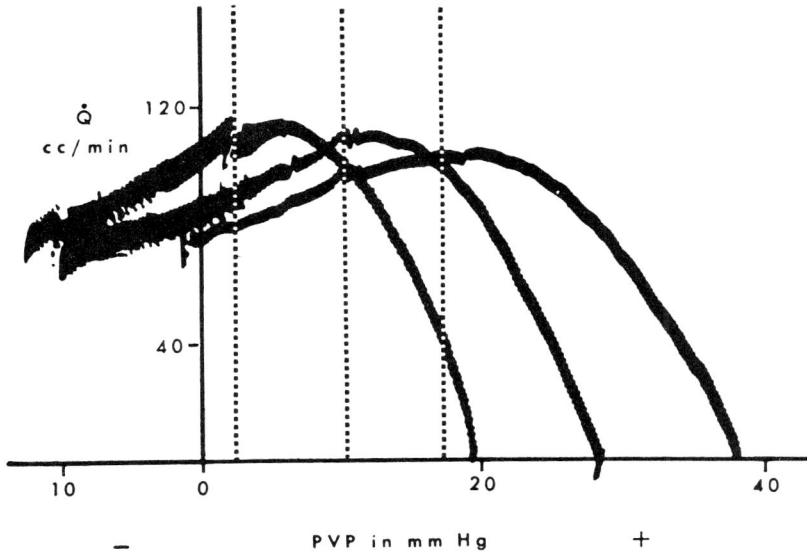

Fig. 21. Pressure-flow relationships of the pulmonary capillaries. (From Permutt, Bromberger, and Bane.[27] Reproduced here with the permission of the publishers.)

lation in normal humans has been provided by West and colleagues.[37,38] These investigators used radioactive isotopes to measure ventilation and blood flow in different regions from top to bottom of the upright human lung. Both pulmonary arterial and venous pressures increase from superior to dependent regions of the lung because of the hydrostatic effect resulting from gravity.* In a typical human lung 30 cm in height the pulmonary artery pressure may be 20 cm H_2O and the pulmonary venous pressure 10 cm H_2O at the most dependent portion of the lung (the diaphragmatic surface). One-third up the lung the pulmonary venous pressure falls to atmospheric pressure; two-thirds up the lung pulmonary artery pressure falls to atmospheric pressure. The alveolar pressure, however, remains essentially constant throught the lung.

*The increase in blood pressure due to gravity is equal to ρgh, where ρ = density of blood (1.05 gm/cm³), g = gravity acceleration constant (980 cm/sec²), and h = vertical distance down the lung. Since ρ and g are constants and the density of blood is approximately that of water, the blood pressure will increase approximately 1 cm H_2O for each cm distance moved down the lung.

This distribution of pressures results in the distribution of blood flow within the lungs to essentially three major zones, depending upon the magnitudes of the pressures. In the upper third of the lung (Zone 1) the alveolar pressure is greater than or equal to pulmonary artery pressure, and there is no flow. In the middle zone (Zone II, the Starling resistor zone) pulmonary arterial pressure is greater than alveolar pressure which is greater than pulmonary venous pressure. In Zone II flow through the pulmonary capillaries is proportional to the difference between pulmonary arterial and alveolar pressure. In Zone III, the dependent region, pulmonary arterial pressure is greater than pulmonary venous pressure which is also greater than alveolar pressure, and alveolar pressure has no influence on flow. Thus we can see there are three major blood flow zones which correspond roughly to the three possible pressure-flow conditions

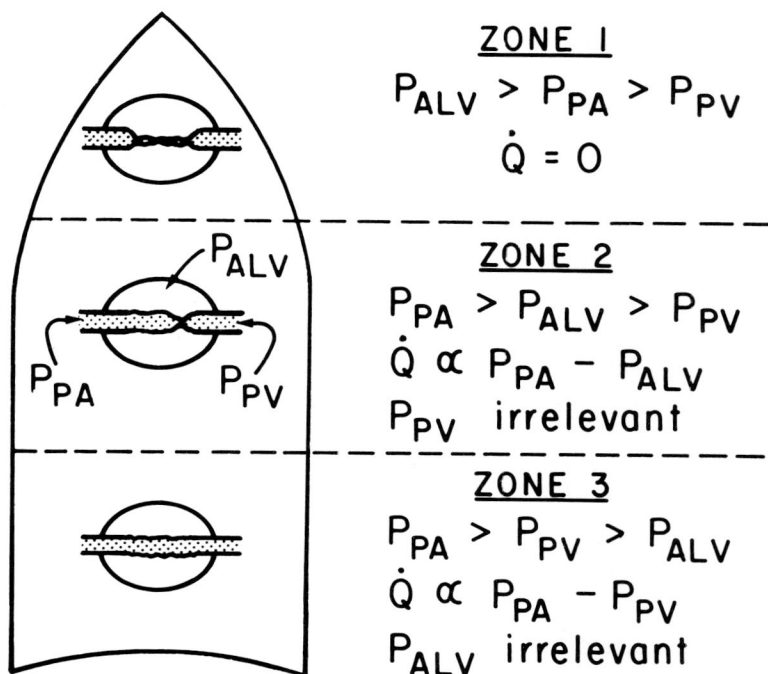

$$\text{ZONE I}$$
$$P_{ALV} > P_{PA} > P_{PV}$$
$$\dot{Q} = 0$$

$$\text{ZONE 2}$$
$$P_{PA} > P_{ALV} > P_{PV}$$
$$\dot{Q} \propto P_{PA} - P_{ALV}$$
$$P_{PV} \text{ irrelevant}$$

$$\text{ZONE 3}$$
$$P_{PA} > P_{PV} > P_{ALV}$$
$$\dot{Q} \propto P_{PA} - P_{PV}$$
$$P_{ALV} \text{ irrelevant}$$

Fig. 22.   Schematic drawing of the three zones of West. P_{PA} = pulmonary arterial pressure, P_{ALV} = alveolar pressure, P_{PV} = pulmonary venous pressure, and $\dot{Q}$ = regional pulmonary blood flow. (From Green, J. F.: The pulmonary circulation. In *The Peripheral Circulations* (R. Zelis, Ed.). New York, Grune & Stratton, 1975. Reproduced here with permission of the publishers.)

of a collapsible tube as discussed above. It is worth mentioning that in the normal upright human lung there is no Zone I, although this condition can develop if pulmonary arterial pressure falls or alveolar pressure rises. Figure 22 is a schematic drawing of the three zones of West; compare each zone with its hydrodynamic equivalent depicted in Figure 7.

Blood flow increases toward the dependent regions of both Zones II and III (Fig. 22). The mechanism for this increase is currently not completely understood. A major cause for the increase in blood flow down Zone II must be related to the increase in the pressure gradient for flow toward the dependent regions of Zone II. The pressure gradient for flow in Zone II is the pulmonary arterial pressure minus the alveolar pressure. Alveolar pressure is constant throughout the zone, but pulmonary arterial pressure increases, because of the hydrostatic effects, toward the dependent regions of the lung. Thus, the pressure gradient increases down Zone II.

This mechanism cannot account for the increase in blood flow down Zone III. The pressure gradient for flow in this zone is the pulmonary artery pressure minus the pulmonary venous pressure, and both pulmonary arterial and venous pressures increase the same amount toward the dependent regions of Zone III (1 cm H_2O per cm distance down the lung). Thus, the pressure gradient ($P_{PA} - P_{PV}$) remains constant in Zone III. The increase in blood flow toward the dependent regions of Zone III is attributed to a constantly decreasing pulmonary vascular resistance. As yet unsettled is the mechanism for this decrease in resistance. Two hypotheses have been proposed (Fig. 23): distension of existing flow channels[37] and recruitment of additional channels.[25]

The *distension hypothesis* makes use of the fact that even though the pressure gradient does not change in Zone III the transmural pressure increases toward the dependent regions of this zone. An increasing transmural pressure should cause an increase in the radius of the pulmonary capillaries, decreasing their resistance. The *recruitment hypothesis* suggests that there is a spectrum of critical opening pressures within the pulmonary vasculature and implies that the pulmonary arterial pressure has to rise above the opening pressure of an individual vessel to allow it to be perfused. There is a higher pulmonary artery pressure at the more dependent regions of the lung; therefore, a greater number of vessels are perfused. This would reduce the pulmonary vascular resistance. Recent evidence[14] suggests that recruitment occurs predominantly under conditions where pulmonary venous pressure is less than alveolar pressure, and

DISTENSION   RECRUITMENT
HYPOTHESIS   HYPOTHESIS

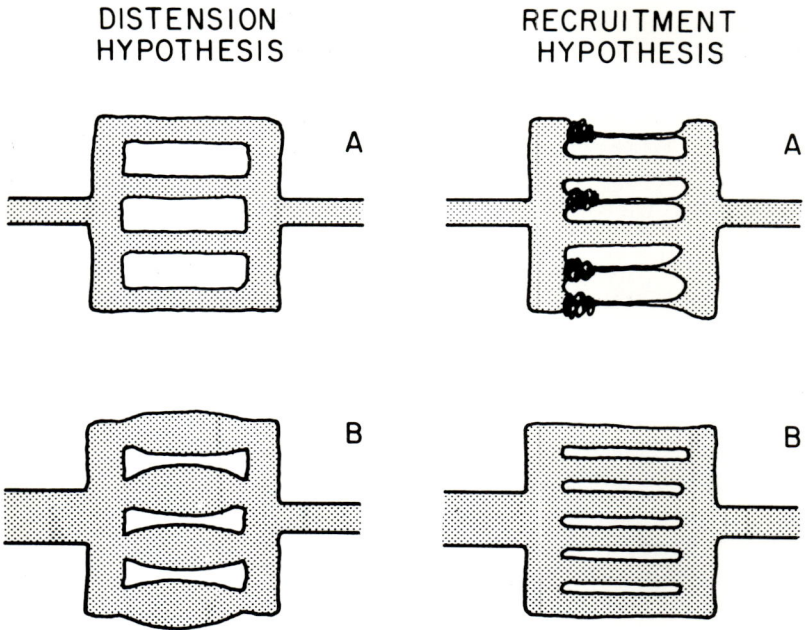

Fig. 23. Schematic drawing representing the two proposed mechanisms for the decreasing vascular resistance down Zone III. *A:* A portion of the pulmonary vasculature toward the top of Zone III. *B:* A portion of the pulmonary vasculature toward the dependent region of Zone III. (From Green, J. F.: The pulmonary circulation. In: *The Peripheral Circulations* (R. Zelis, Ed.). New York, Grune & Stratton, 1975. Reproduced here with permission of the publishers.)

distension occurs predominantly under conditions where pulmonary venous pressure is greater than alveolar pressure. Thus, recruitment and the increasing pressure gradient may account for the increase in blood flow down Zone II, whereas distension may account for the increase in blood flow down Zone III. Undoubtedly we have not heard the last about why blood flow increases toward the dependent regions of the lung.

PULMONARY VASCULAR RESISTANCE

The resistance of the pulmonary vasculature is conventionally calculated as the difference between pulmonary arterial pressure and left atrial pressure divided by the cardiac output. The implicit assumption in this calculation is that left atrial pressure is the effective back pressure for blood flow through the lungs. With the recognition that, under Zone II conditions, alveolar pressure and not pulmonary venous pressure is the back pressure, some investigators have questioned the meaning of pulmonary vascular resistance as conventionally calculated.[27] An increase in the ratio of driving pressure to flow merely indicates that something has happened within the vascular bed somewhere between the points where the pressures were measured to cause an increase in the amount of potential energy dissipated. Given laminar flow and constant blood viscosity and vessel lengths, a change in pulmonary vascular resistance calculated using left atrial pressure as back pressure can only be interpreted as evidence of a change in total vascular cross-section somewhere in the pulmonary vascular bed, as Poiseuille's law (Appendix I) implies, but the cause and site of this change cannot be determined from such a measurement.[26] However, under Zone II conditions (Fig. 21), inferences can be drawn concerning arterial diameter and some undetermined proximal part of the capillary bed if alveolar pressure is substituted for left atrial pressure in the resistance formula. Thus, in order to be able to interpret measurements of pulmonary vascular resistance correctly, one must know the zonal conditions under which the measurements were made and must also use the appropriate back pressure in the resistance formula.

THE EFFECT OF LUNG INFLATION ON PULMONARY PRESSURE-FLOW RELATIONSHIPS

Lung inflation affects the pressure-flow relationships of the pulmonary vasculature both directly, by compressing the small vessels, and indirectly, through the effect of pleural pressure on venous return and pulmonary blood flow. We shall first consider the direct effect of lung inflation per se by considering the pulmonary blood flow constant.

An increase in lung volume necessitates an increase in transpulmonary pressure (the difference between alveolar pressure and pleural pressure, Chap. 10). This may be accomplished by either a decrease in pleural pressure relative to atmospheric pressure (spontaneous respiration) or an increase in alveolar pressure relative to atmospheric pressure (positive pressure respiration). Left atrial pressure relative to pleural pressure tends to remain constant at constant cardiac output (Chap. 8). Thus, an increase in lung volume which necessitates an increase in alveolar pressure relative to pleural pressure results in an increase in alveolar pressure relative to left atrial pressure. This will occur regardless of whether the lung is inflated by spontaneous respiration or by positive pressure ventilation. Lung inflation, therefore, causes the small alveolar vessels (those directly exposed to alveolar pressure) to be compressed. The end-result is an increase in that portion of the lung in Zone II and an increase in the resistance to flow in all vessels exposed to alveolar pressure.

Pulmonary vascular resistance increases not only at high states of lung inflation but also at low levels of inflation.[21,22] There is, thus, a U-shaped curve of pulmonary vascular resistance versus lung inflation. The high vascular resistance at low states of lung inflation is probably caused by narrowing of extra-alveolar vessels, those arteries and veins which are not directly exposed to alveolar pressure and which run though the lung parenchyma. The caliber of extra-alveolar vessels is affected by lung volume; decreasing lung volume decreases the radius of extra-alveolar vessels, increasing the pulmonary vascular resistance.

The pulmonary vasculature is also influenced by the effect that lung inflation has upon venous return. During a spontaneous respiration, right atrial pressure falls with pleural pressure. The fall in right atrial pressure increases venous return which, when passed on to the lungs, causes a fall in pulmonary vascular resistance by one of the possible mechanisms discussed above. With positive pressure ventilation, right atrial pressure rises, venous return falls, and pulmonary vascular resistances increase. Thus, the rise in pulmonary vascular resistance by compression of the small alveolar vessels with spontaneous inspiration tends to be negated by the increases in venous return, whereas with positive pressure ventilation it tends to be accentuated by the fall in venous return. Overdistension of the lungs during positive pressure breathing, therefore, results in an increase in the amount of work the right ventricle has to do to pump the same amount of blood and so can be associated with harmful consequences, particularly in patients who have pre-existing impairment of right ventricular function.

PULMONARY VENOUS RETURN

In Chapter 5 the pressure-flow relationship through the systemic venous system was described by the following expression:

$$\dot{Q}_S = \frac{P_{MS} - P_{RA}}{R_{VS}}, \qquad (11)$$

where $\dot{Q}_S$ = systemic venous return, P_{MS} = mean systemic pressure (pressure within the compliant area of the systemic circulation), P_{RA} = right atrial pressure, and R_{VS} = resistance of the veins between the compliant areas and the right atrium, i.e. the systemic venous resistance. This pressure-flow relationship was the inevitable consequence of the structure of the systemic venous system in which the major compliant areas are upstream from the small but significant resistance to venous return. Evidence also suggests that the same condition exists in the pulmonary circulation. It has been shown[13] that approximately 45 per cent of the total pulmonary vascular compliance is located at the level of the small pulmonary veins, whereas the compliance of the large pulmonary veins accounts for only 15 per cent of the distribution of the total pulmonary vascular compliance; the remaining compliance is divided about equally among large arteries, small arteries, and capillaries. This allows us to consider pulmonary venous return ($\dot{Q}_P$) with the aid of the same type of conceptual model we used with systemic venous return:

$$\dot{Q}_P = \frac{P_{MP} - P_{LA}}{R_{VP}}, \tag{20}$$

where P_{MP} = mean pulmonary pressure (pressure within the compliant areas of the pulmonary circulation), P_{LA} = left atrial pressure, and R_{VS} = the resistance of the veins between the compliant areas of the pulmonary vascular bed and the left atrium, i.e. the pulmonary venous resistance.

The important parameters for the systemic and pulmonary venous systems are compared in Table 3. Immediately apparent is the gross disparity between the compliances. The systemic compliance is approximately 12 times greater than the pulmonary. The significance of this was discussed in Chapter 3. In brief, it means the pulmonary vessels cannot be a significant vascular reservoir. The next most obvious dissimilarity between

Table 3. Comparison of the Circulatory Parameters for the Systemic and Pulmonary Vascular Beds

C_S	C_P	P_S	P_P	P_{RA}	P_{LA}	R_{VS}	R_{VP}	$\dot{Q}_S$	$\dot{Q}_P$
($ml \cdot mmHg^{-1} \cdot kg^{-1}$)		(mm Hg)				($mmHg \cdot l^{-1} \cdot min$)		(l/min)	
2.6	0.2	7.0	5.0	0	4.0	4.4	0.6	1.6	1.6

the greater and lesser circulations is the venous resistances. The pulmonary venous resistance is only one-seventh that of the systemic venous resistance. This would suggest, as is the case, a very small pressure drop (1 mm Hg) between the primary capacitance areas, immediately downstream from the capillaries and the left atrium.

In summary, the pulmonary capillaries are collapsible vessels which function as Starling resistors whenever pulmonary venous pressure is less than alveolar pressure. The compliance of the pulmonary circulation is considerably less than that of the systemic circulation; thus, the pulmonary circulation cannot be a significant vascular reservoir.

8

Pressure-flow Relationships of the Heart

DETERMINANTS OF FLOW THROUGH THE HEART

The *cardiac output* is the amount of blood pumped by the heart per unit of time. Anything that alters venous return will alter cardiac output. Therefore, under normal conditions the determinants of cardiac output are essentially the determinants of venous return which are discussed in Chapter 5. This statement assumes a normal healthy heart capable of simply passing on to the arteries the blood the veins return to it. In this chapter we will consider how the heart passes on the venous return. In other words, we will consider the determinants of flow through the heart.

The amount of blood that the heart pumps is equal to the stroke volume times the heart rate. The stroke volume is the amount of blood (ml) per beat that the heart pumps, and the heart rate is the number of beats per minute. As venous return is changed the cardiac output is adjusted by changing either the stroke volume or the frequency, or both. An adjustment of heart rate usually results from reflexes initiated from the systemic circulation. However, the ability to change stroke volume is an inherent property of the heart muscle and can occur even with total denervation of the heart.

The basic mechanism of adjusting stroke volume has been described by *Starling's law of the heart* (also known as the Frank-Starling relationship). Briefly, Starling's law states that

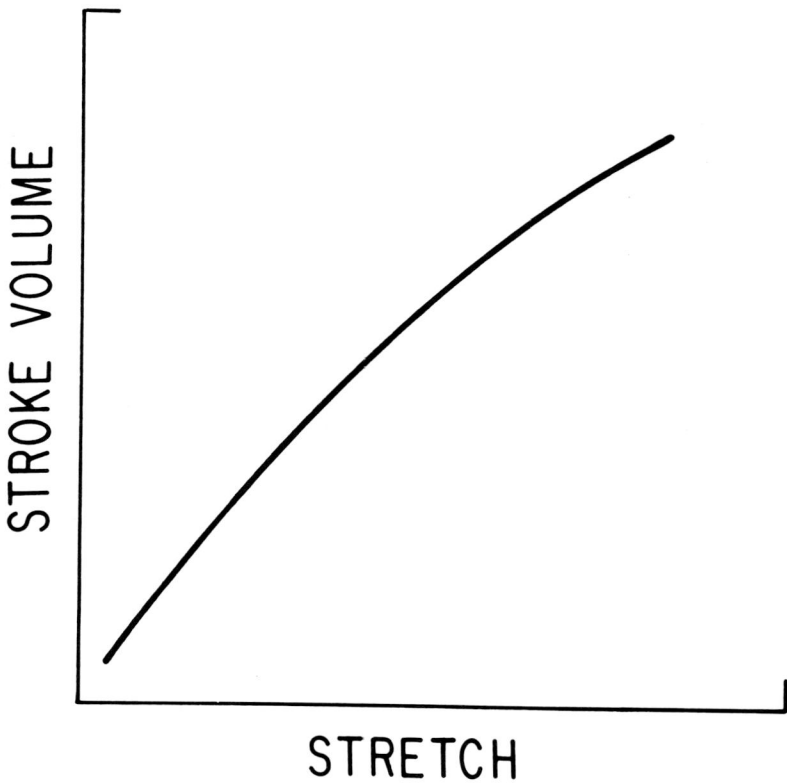

Fig. 24. The Frank-Starling relationship—stroke volume as a function of ventricular end-diastolic stretch. An increase in the stretch of the ventricles immediately before contraction (end-diastole) results in an increase in stroke volume.

an increase in the stretch of the ventricles immediately before contraction (end-diastole) results in an increase in stroke volume. Since it is difficult to quantitate directly the amount of ventricular stretch, indirect measurements of stretch are made. These include ventricular end-diastolic volume, ventricular end-diastolic transmural pressure, or transmural atrial pressure. Figure 24 shows the type of relationship obtained when stroke volume is plotted against some index of ventricular end-diastolic stretch. An increase in stretch increases ventricular performance. Such a relationship is generally referred to as a ventricular or cardiac function curve.

Although a stroke volume function curve may be adequate for describing the heart's ability to pump a certain amount of blood per beat, its usefulness is limited. Other indexes of ventricular performance such as stroke work, minute work, or cardiac output are often more informative, especially if we wish to assess the pumping ability of the heart over a period of time. If we wanted to study the heart's ability to pump the venous return we would select cardiac output as the index of ventricular performance. If, on the other hand, we were interested in the amount of work the heart could do we would use stroke work or minute work as an index of ventricular performance. A commonly used cardiac output function curve is shown in Figure 25. Right atrial transmural pressure is used as the index of ventricular stretch. The reasoning goes as follows: the greater the right atrial transmural pressure, the greater is the ventricular filling, the greater the

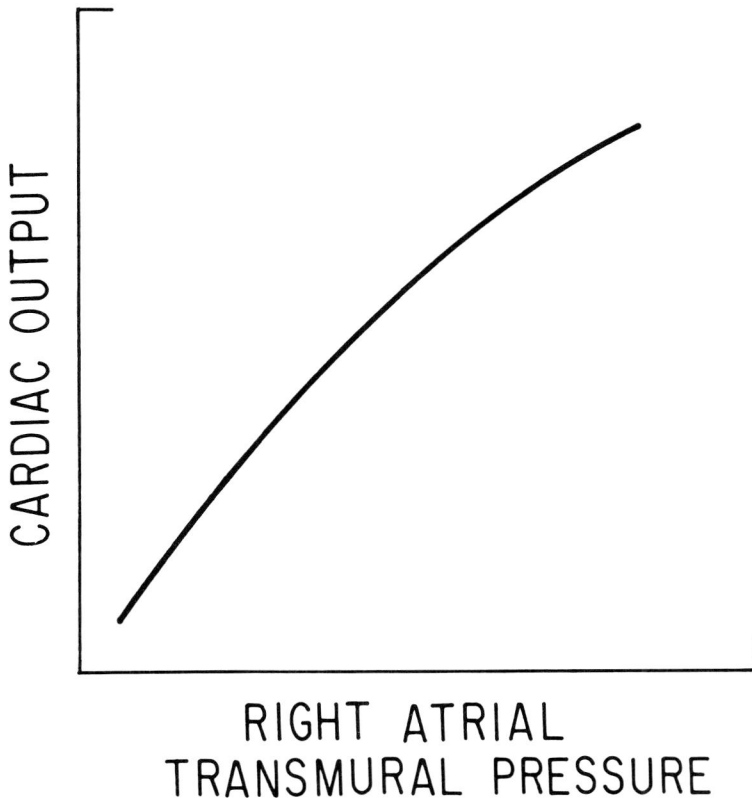

Fig. 25. A right ventricular cardiac function curve. An increase in the right atrial pressure results in an increase in right ventricular stretch, then ventricular (cardiac) output. This relationship assumes heart rate is constant.

end-diastolic volume, the greater is the ventricular stretch. If the heart rate remains constant, the increased cardiac output results solely from the increased ventricular stretch.

PATTERNS OF VENTRICULAR PERFORMANCE

It should be obvious that an infinite number of cardiac function curves are possible. At any given degree of stretch a normal heart should be able to pump more blood and do more work than a *hypoeffective* heart (i.e. diseased heart). Similarly a *hypereffective* heart should give a better performance than a normal heart.

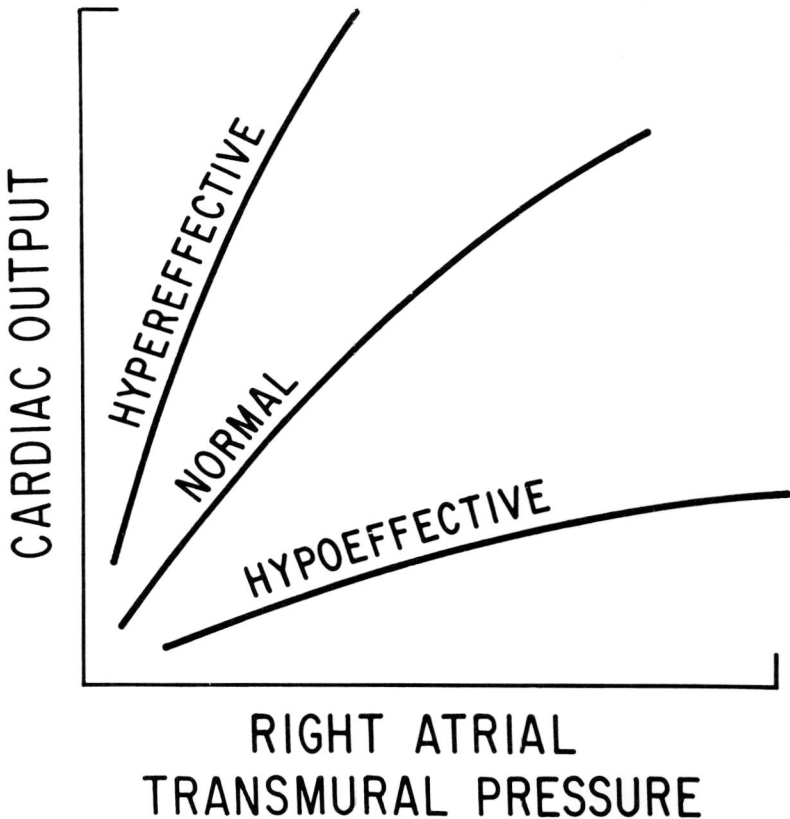

Fig. 26.   Basic patterns of ventricular function curves. For a hypereffective heart a given increase in right atrial pressure results in a greater than normal increase in cardiac output. For a hypoeffective heart the same increase in right atrial pressure results in a less than normal increase in cardiac output.

Figure 26 demonstrates the basic patterns of cardiac function curves. The slope of the cardiac function curve is a function of the inherent property of the myocardium. The term *contractility* is usually applied to describe the state of the myocardium. An increased contractility produces a hypereffective heart and increases the slope of the cardiac function curve. A decrease in contractility produces a hypoeffective heart and decreases the slope of the curve. Factors which can lead to a hypereffective heart are increased sympathetic nerve activity to the heart, an increase in the level of circulating catecholamines, or the administration of an exogenous positive inotropic agent, e.g. one which strengthens muscular action, such as the cardiac glycosides and isoproterenol. Factors which can lead to a hypoeffective heart are decreased sympathetic nerve activity to the heart, physiologic depressants (such as myocardial hypoxia, hypercapnia, and acidosis), pharmacologic depressants (such as barbiturates), and loss of myocardium, as that which occurs following an infarction.

In summary, the determinants of flow through the heart consist of those factors which control heart rate and stroke volume, the latter being determined by the contractility of the myocardium and the degree of stretch of the ventricles.

9

Practical Aspects of Circulatory Mechanics

In previous chapters the basic concepts used to describe the mechanical properties of the circulatory system were discussed and a conceptual model of the circulatory system was developed. The object of this chapter is to demonstrate how the conceptual model of the circulatory system can be used to understand the control of cardiac output.

DUALITY OF CARDIAC OUTPUT CONTROL

In many respects the terms *cardiac output* and *venous return* are unfortunate semantic choices because they suggest entirely different flows, but, as we have seen, because of the closed and circular nature of the cardiovascular system, they must remain equal except for minor transient periods.* Therefore, it should be obvious that both the circuit and the heart should play important roles in determining the total systemic flow. Since there is a natural inclination to associate cardiac output control with the heart, most physiologists are unaware of the contribution made by the systemic blood vessels, despite much important and significant work.[8,19,36,24] Nevertheless, cardiac output control rests as much with systemic factors as with cardiac factors. The reason for this, as succinctly stated by Grodins,[18] is that ". . . mechanical coupling between heart and circuit dictates that cardiac output is a function of both heart and circuit parame-

---

*Perhaps a better choice of terms would be *total systemic flow*.

71

ters." A full appreciation of this statement is indispensable in understanding the operation of the cardiovascular system.

Right Atrial Pressure as a Coupler

The right atrial pressure is a unique pressure in the cardio-vascular system. It is not only the back pressure to the systemic circulation but also the simultaneous inflow pressure for the heart. The right atrial pressure is, thus, a function of the amount of blood returned to the heart and the pumping ability of the heart. If the heart were a perfect pump, the right atrial pressure would always be maintained at an atmospheric or slightly subatmospheric value. This would establish a maximum gradient for venous return. If the heart were anything less than a perfect pump, the right atrial pressure would rise to a positive value thereby reducing the pressure gradient for venous return. In essence, the right atrial pressure couples the pumping ability of the heart to the systemic circulation by directly affecting the pressure gradient for venous return. Such mechanical coupling between heart and circuit is absolutely essential if cardiac output is to remain equal to venous return.

The coupling nature of the right atrial pressure is best seen with the aid of the cardiac function and venous return curves. Figure 27a presents a cardiac function curve with right atrial pressure measured relative to atmospheric pressure as the independent variable. (This figure, as well as all subsequent ones, was originally obtained from animal experiments[19] and extrapolated to the human.) The magnitude of the right atrial pressure at zero cardiac output is equal to the pleural pressure, for it is at this point that the transmural pressure is zero. A venous return curve, identical to those discussed earlier (Chap. 5) is presented in Figure 27b. The cardiac function curve represents all possible combinations of cardiac output and right atrial pressure. The venous return curve represents all possible combinations of venous return and right atrial pressure. At any one moment under steady-state conditions there is one and only one cardiac output which must be equal to venous return and one and only one right atrial pressure. The exact combination of flow and right atrial pressure can be obtained by combining the cardiac function curve and venous return curve on the same axes. This was done in Figure 27c and represents a graphic analysis of the determinants of cardiac output. Given any constant blood volume, systemic compliance, venous resistance, cardiac contractility, and pleural pressure, the resulting cardiac

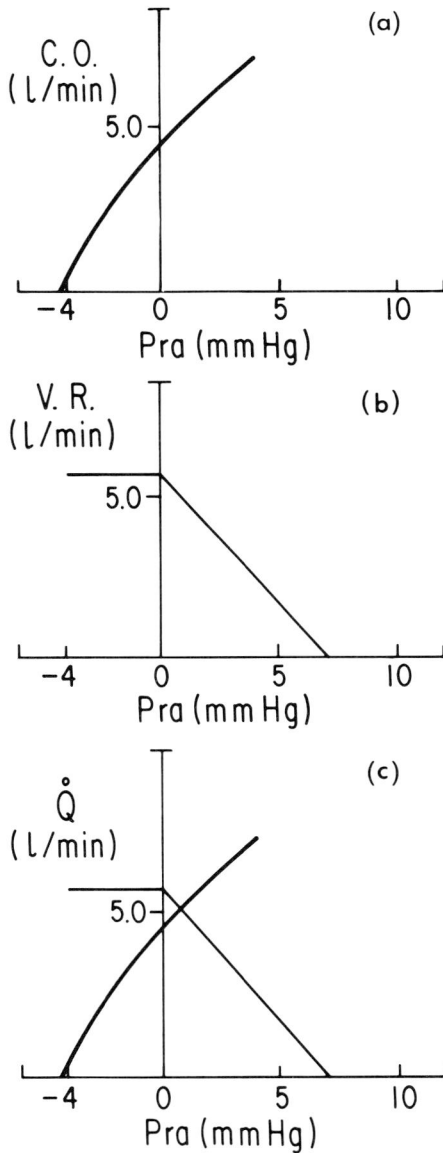

Fig. 27. a: Cardiac function curve—cardiac output as a function of right atrial pressure, measured relative to atmospheric pressure. b: Venous return curve—venous return as a function of right atrial pressure, measured relative to atmospheric pressure. The cardiac function curve represents all possible combinations of cardiac output and right atrial pressure. The venous return curve represents all possible combinations of venous return and right atrial pressure. Since cardiac output and venous return must be equal there can only be one possible combination of total systemic flow ($\dot{Q}$) and right atrial pressure. This can be determined by the intersection of the cardiac function and venous return curves when plotted on the same coordinates (c).

output, venous return, and right atrial pressure may be determined by the intersection of the cardiac function and venous return curves.

CARDIAC FACTORS INFLUENCING VENOUS RETURN

Figure 28 presents a graphic analysis with three function curves corresponding to the normal, hypoeffective, and hyper-effective heart, and further illustrates the coupling nature of the right atrial pressure. Point A represents a normal cardiac output of 5 l/min and a right atrial pressure of about 1 mm Hg. Blood is returned to the heart with a pressure gradient ($P_{MS} - P_{RA}$) of 6 mm Hg. If the heart were to suddenly become hypoeffective without any significant changes in the systemic blood vessels it would be unable to pump 5 l/min. There would be a brief period where venous inflow to the heart would exceed the heart's ability to remove blood from the veins. Right atrial pressure would rise until the pressure gradient for venous return (3 mm Hg) reduced venous return to match cardiac output. The circulation would

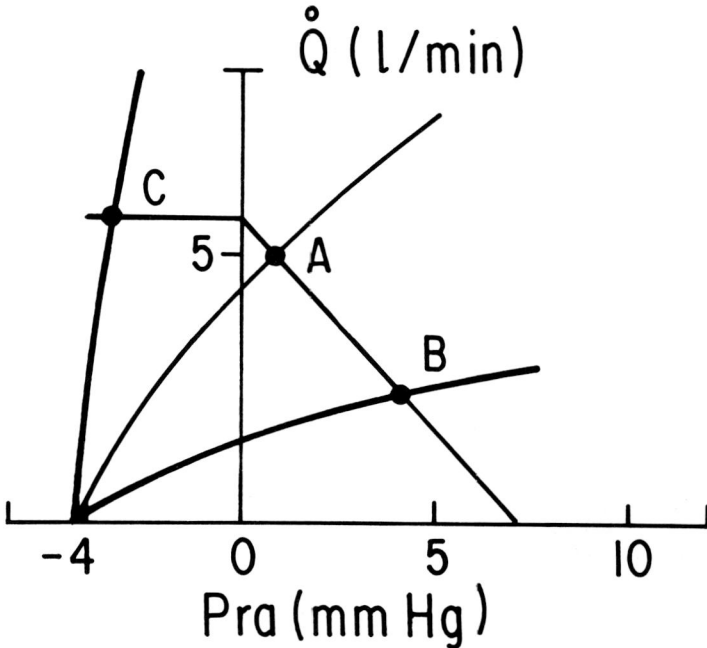

Fig. 28. Graphic analysis of the cardiovascular system illustrating the effect of a normal (A), hypoeffective (B), and hypereffective (C) heart.

once again be in balance, and the steady-state cardiac function curve would have moved from point A to point B along the venous return curve (Fig. 28). The rise in right atrial pressure serves to couple the venous return to cardiac output. If the heart's pumping ability suddenly increased it could not actually pump more blood unless the venous return increased. The increased pumping action of the heart lowers right atrial pressure which increases the pressure gradient ($P_{MS} - P_{RA}$) and increases venous return. Further decreases in P_{RA} will continue to produce further increases in venous return until P_{RA} falls below atmospheric pressure, at which point collapse of the great veins occurs, and venous return becomes fixed at its maximum pressure gradient (7 mm Hg). At point C, the heart potentially could pump more blood than it does. This is a perfect example of the truism, "The heart cannot pump more blood than it receives." To increase cardiac output under these conditions (curve C) the systemic factors influencing venous return must actively change.

SYSTEMIC FACTORS INFLUENCING CARDIAC OUTPUT

Until now we have considered only how cardiac output could be varied by changing cardiac factors (inotropic and chronotropic properties of the heart) while maintaining circuit parameters (volume, compliance, etc.) constant. We will now consider how cardiac output can be varied by altering circuit parameters while keeping cardiac factors constant. Figure 29 presents a graphic analysis of the circulatory system with three different venous return curves representing a normal (A), increased (B), and decreased (C) mean systemic pressure. If the mean systemic pressure were suddenly increased from its normal value of 7.0 mm Hg to 12.0 mm Hg, venous return would increase, raising right atrial pressure. The rise in right atrial pressure would increase the filling of the heart, stretching the ventricles, and through the Starling mechanism increase cardiac output to match the venous return. The venous return curve would shift to the right, changing the intersection with the ventricular function curve from point A to point B. A reduction in mean systemic pressure would shift the venous return curve to the left, intersecting the cardiac function curve at point C. In these examples right atrial pressure also served as the coupling mechanism between venous return and cardiac output.

From the preceding illustration it should be obvious that the control of cardiac output does not rest exclusively with heart factors but also with systemic ones. Consider the important exam-

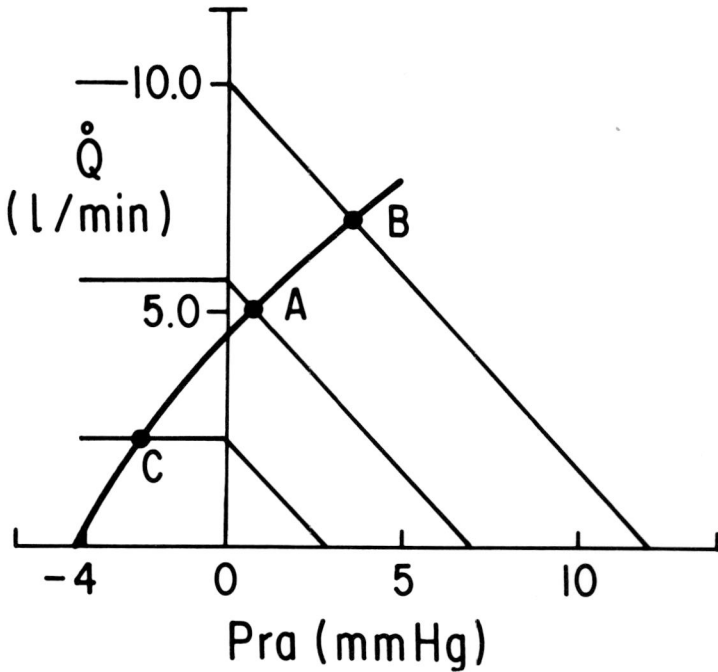

Fig. 29. Graphic analysis of the cardiovascular system illustrating the effect of a normal (A), increased (B), and decreased (C) mean systemic pressure.

ple of exercise. Exercise is known to increase the cardiac output from the normal resting value of 5 l/min to well over 25 l/min. If the inotropic and chronotropic properties of the heart were the only factors to change during exercise, cardiac output would not significantly increase. The normal right atrial pressure is only about 1 mm Hg. Increasing the pumping ability of the heart would lower right pressure, but as soon as the right atrial pressure was reduced to atmospheric pressure the veins entering the chest would collapse, limiting the venous return. This can be seen in Figure 30. If only cardiac factors were operative in exercise, the equilibrium point would move only from A on the normal curve to B, increasing cardiac output by only a few hundred cc per min. To significantly increase cardiac output there must also be active changes on the part of the systemic blood vessels, i.e. a decrease in systemic compliance or venous resistance. In other words, to get a fivefold increase in cardiac output it is not enough to augment the slope of the cardiac function curve. The venous return curve must

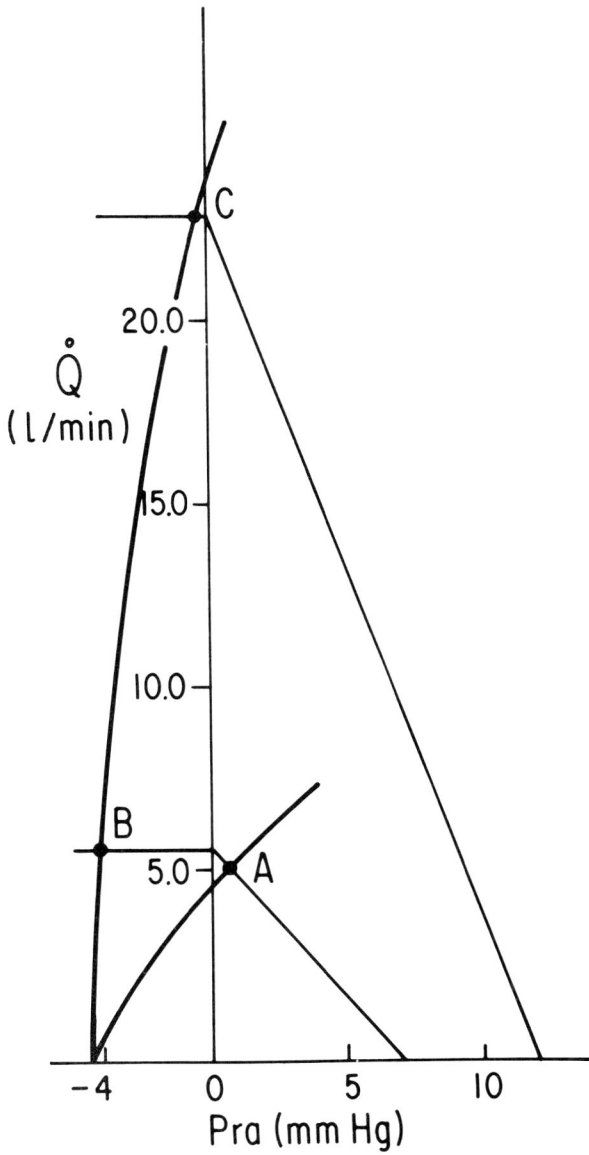

Fig. 30. Graphic analysis of the cardiovascular system illustrating response to exercise. See text for details.

also shift to the right and increase its slope, shifting the equilibrium point from A to C (Fig. 30).

THE CONTROLLING MECHANISMS OF CARDIAC OUTPUT

A few words are now in order concerning the mechanisms responsible for changes in mean systemic pressure, the resistance to venous return, and the contractile properties of the heart. These mechanisms are responsible for the shape and position of the venous return and cardiac function curves. The parameters which affect the mean systemic pressure are essentially those which determine the static volume-pressure relationship of the systemic circulation (Chaps. 1 and 3), the stressed volume (V), the unstressed volume (V_0), and the compliance (C). The most immediate way to increase or decrease V is by transfusion or hemorrhage. C and V_0 can be indirectly changed through reflex adjustment of vascular smooth muscle tone or directly altered by direct stimulation of the vascular smooth muscle by such agents as epinephrine or exogenous drugs. R_V can similarly be changed by indirect reflex adjustment and direct chemical stimulation. In addition, R_V can be altered by changes in the transmural pressure of the venous resistance vessels, which usually occur because of volume shifts into and out of these vessels. Changes in cardiac parameters sufficient to alter the slope of the cardiac function curve are usually those which alter the inotropic and chronotropic properties of the myocardium (Chap. 8). The cardiac function curve is shifted along the pressure axes by changes in pleural pressure.

In summary, cardiac output is controlled not only by how well the heart is able to pump blood but also by the ability of the systemic blood vessels to return blood to the heart. To have a significant increase in cardiac output, as that which occurs during exercise, there must be active alterations in both heart and circuit parameters.

SECTION III:

PULMONARY MECHANICS

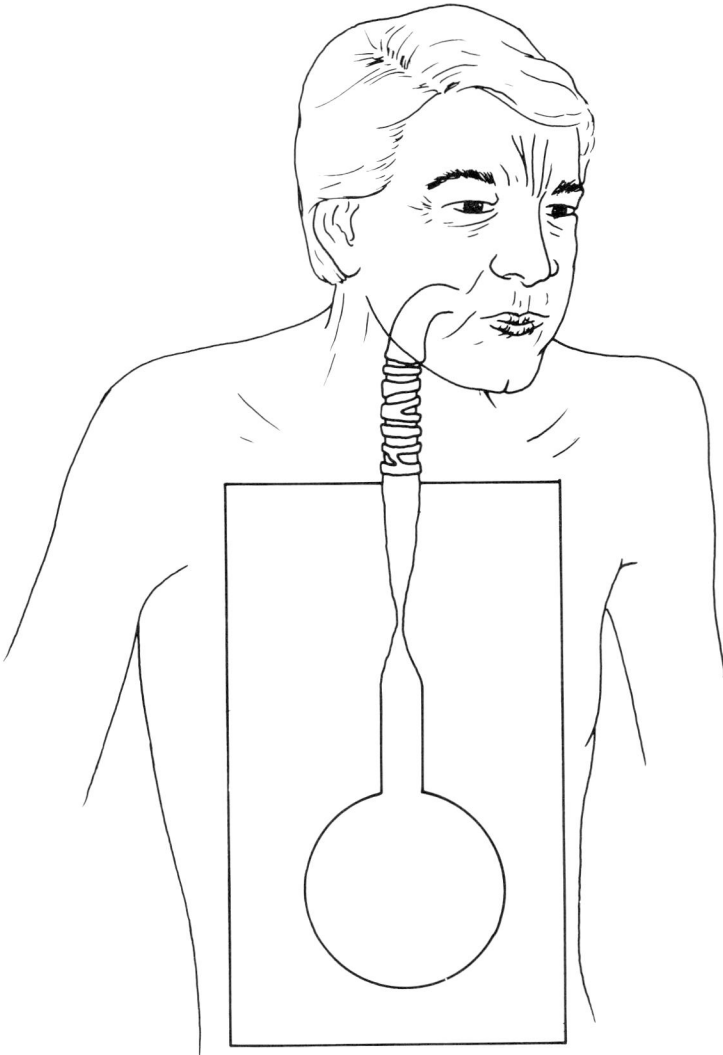

10

Volume-pressure Relationships of the Lung

PULMONARY (ALVEOLAR) COMPLIANCE

The relationship of a change in lung volume to a change in distending pressure of the lungs is the compliance of the lungs, and is determined by their elastic properties. The elasticity of the lungs is derived essentially from two sources: elastic elements within the lungs and the surface tension of the thin layer of fluid which lines the alveoli. Abnormalities in either of these elastic sources can alter pulmonary compliance and interfere with normal functioning of the lungs.

Since the lungs are elastic, an increase in their volume is dependent upon an increase in their transmural pressure (distending pressure). The transmural pressure of the lungs is called the *transpulmonary pressure* and is the difference between the pressure inside the lungs, the alveolar pressure (P_A), and the pressure at the outer surface of the lungs. Under normal conditions when the lungs are within the chest cavity, the pressure at the outer surface of the lungs is the pleural pressure (P_{PL}); however, when the chest is open, the pressure at the outer surface of the lungs is atmospheric pressure (P_{ATM}, considered zero).* The transpulmonary pressure (P_{TP}) may be summarized as:

$$P_{TP} = P_A - P_{PL}, \text{ normal conditions}$$
$$P_{TP} = P_A - P_{ATM} = P_A, \text{ chest open} \tag{21}$$

---

*For convenience, the atmospheric pressure is always considered to be zero. The measured values for P_A and P_{PL} under different circumstances, thus, denote the change (increase or decrease) in pressure ($\triangle P$) from P_{ATM}.

Since there are two determinants of the transpulmonary pressure under normal conditions, there are two ways of increasing the lung volume: either by increasing the pressure inside the lung relative to that at the surface (increasing P_A relative to P_{PL}) or by decreasing the pressure at the surface relative to that inside (decreasing P_{PL} relative to P_A). The former situation occurs during positive pressure respiration and is used by the anesthesiologist to ventilate a paralyzed patient. The latter circumstance occurs during normal spontaneous breathing. With an open chest, the only way lung volume can be increased is by positive pressure ventilation. Thus, a patient undergoing thoracic surgery is ventilated in this manner.

Regardless of how the transpulmonary pressure is increased (by positive pressure ventilation or spontaneous inspiration), the increase in lung volume divided by the increased transpulmonary pressure ($\Delta V/\Delta P_{TP}$) defines the compliance. A plot of ΔV against ΔP_{TP} is known as the compliance curve of the lungs, the slope of which is equal to the compliance.* Figure 31 illustrates hypothetical compliance curves of a lung, assuming linear compliance. The straight line represents the pressure-volume relationships that would be obtained under static conditions, that is,

---

*Introduced here is one of the most potentially confusing issues in this book. In Chapter 1, discussing the basics of volume-pressure relationship, a figure was presented of volume plotted on the abscissa and pressure on the ordinant (Fig. 4). Figure 31 presents a plot of pressure on the abscissa and volume on the ordinant and is called a pressure-volume relationship. The important question here is when is volume or pressure plotted on the abscissa? By convention the independent variable is usually thus plotted. To change lung volume, transpulmonary pressure is changed independently and the change in lung volume which results is observed. The final volume is dependent upon the magnitude of the change in transpulmonary pressure. The transpulmonary pressure is plotted on the abscissa and lung volume on the ordinant. In Chapter 1, we talked about changing the volume in hypothetical balloons and observing the resulting change in pressure. That is why volume (the independent variable) was plotted on the abscissa and pressure on the ordinant. In Chapter 3 we discussed compliance curves of the circulatory system. These curves are obtained by changing the blood volume and observing the resulting change in blood pressure. Thus, as in Chapter 1, volume was plotted on the abscissa. If two important facts are remembered, confusion over this convention will be avoided: (1) the independent variable (that which is initially altered) is plotted on the abscissa and (2) the ratio of change in volume over change in pressure is always called the compliance, i.e. $\Delta V/\Delta P = C$. The ratio of the change in pressure over the change in volume is equal to the reciprocal of compliance, i.e. $\Delta P/\Delta V = 1/C$. If one wishes to apply a name to $\Delta P/\Delta V$ it can be called the elastance, although this term is seldom used.

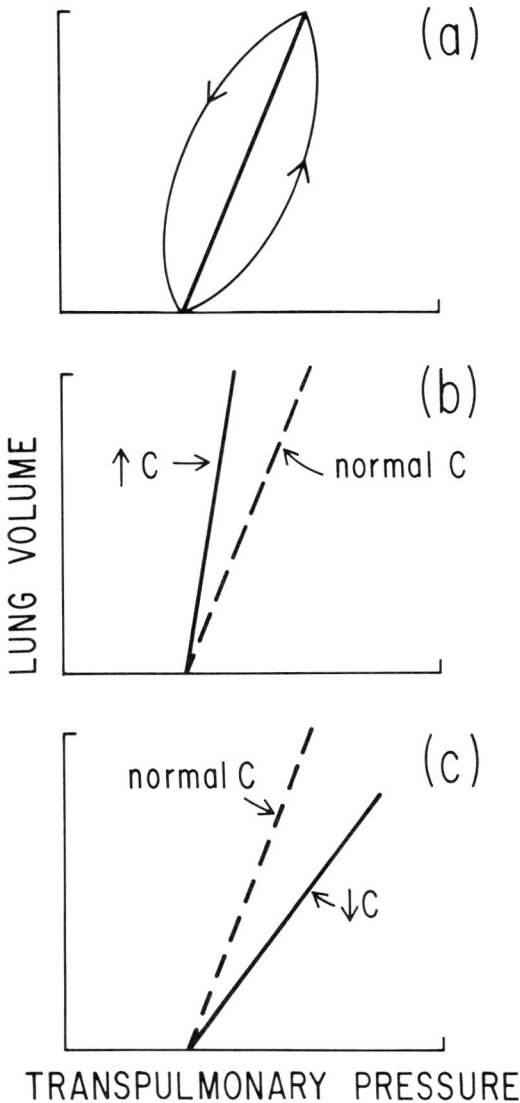

Fig. 31.   *a:* Hypothetical pressure-volume curves of the normal lung. The straight line represents the static pressure-volume relationship. The curved lines represent the pressure-volume relationships obtained under dynamic conditions. *b:* Hypothetical pressure-volume curve of a lung with increased compliance. A lesser pressure change is required to achieve a unit change in volume. *c:* Hypothetical pressure-volume curve of a lung with decreased compliance. A greater pressure change is required to achieve a unit change in volume.

if P_{TP} was increased and held constant until volume stopped changing. The static pressure-volume curve would be the same regardless of whether P_{TP} was increased by increasing P_A relative to P_{PL} or decreasing P_{PL} relative to P_A. It represents the true compliance curve of the lung. The curved lines represent the pressure-volume relationships that would be obtained during a dynamic inspiration and expiration. The horizontal distance at any volume between the dynamic and static curves represents the pressure needed to overcome the resistance to air flow through the lungs (Chap. 11, Fig. 39). The effect of airway resistance on the pressure-volume curves of the lung is introduced here only to demonstrate that lung compliance curves must be obtained under static conditions (when no flow is occurring). For this reason the rest of the discussion of lung compliance will assume static measurements. An increase in lung compliance (a flabby lung) would be manifested as an increase in slope of the pressure-volume relationship, whereas a decrease in lung compliance (a stiff lung) would be indicated by a decrease in the slope of the pressure-volume relationship. Hypothetical compliance curves representing increased and decreased lung compliances, respectively, are presented in Figure 31b,c.

In summary, the ratio of the change in lung volume to change in transpulmonary pressure under static conditions is by definition the compliance of the lung and is an index of lung elasticity. If the lungs are stiff, the ratio is small, and if the lungs are flabby the ratio is large. To say it another way, the static transpulmonary pressure depends only on the volume and the compliance of the lungs.

CHEST WALL COMPLIANCE

The chest wall is also an elastic structure. In a manner analogous to that of the lung, the compliance of the chest wall is defined as the change in thoracic volume divided by the distending pressure of the thorax, P_{CW}. P_{CW} is the difference between the pressure at the inside surface of the chest wall, the pleural pressure, and the pressure at the outside surface of the chest wall, the atmospheric pressure. Thus

$$P_{CW} = P_{PL} - P_{ATM} . \qquad (22)$$

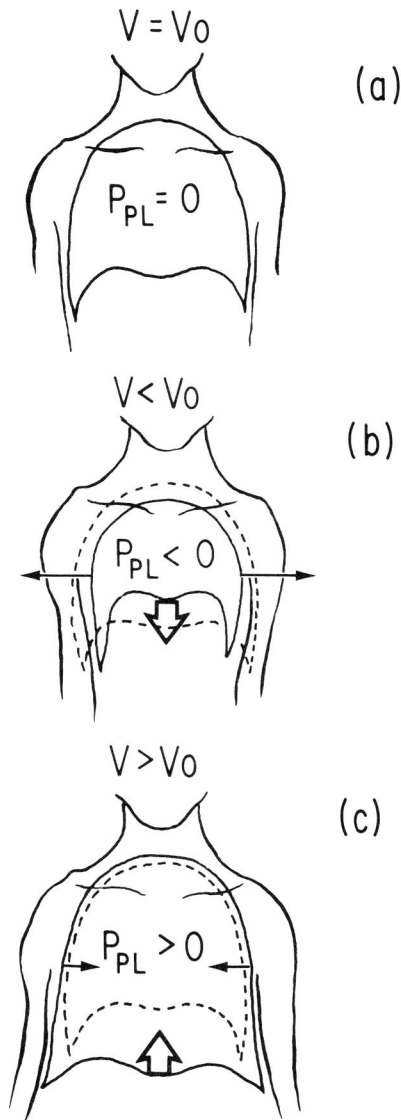

Fig. 32. Chest wall recoil illustrated for three hypothetical situations in which the lungs are absent. *a:* The intrathoracic pressure is atmospheric so that the thoracic volume is equal to the unstressed thoracic volume ($V = V_0$), i.e. there is no deformation of the chest wall so pleural pressure (P_{PL}) is equal to ambiant pressure (0). *b:* Air is removed from the thorax so that thoracic volume is less than the unstressed thoracic volume ($V < V_0$). When $V < V_0$, the chest wall recoils in the outward direction and P_{PL} (intrathoracic pressure) becomes subatmospheric. *c:* Air is forced into the thorax so that thoracic volume is greater than the unstressed thoracic volume ($V > V_0$). When $V > V_0$, the chest wall recoils in the inward direction and pleural pressure becomes greater than atmospheric pressure. The dashed lines represent V_0.

Unlike the lung, which recoils only in the inward direction, the chest wall will recoil either inward or outward depending upon the volume of the chest.

For the purposes of discussing the elastic properties of the chest wall, let us consider the hypothetical thought experiment illustrated by Figure 32. Assume that the thoracic contents (heart, lungs, etc.) have been removed and the chest wall has been sewed up to be air tight. The pressure throughout the empty cavity is still the pressure at the inner surface of the chest wall and as such can be called the pleural pressure. If, under conditions of relaxed respiratory muscles, the volume of the thorax is now adjusted so that the pleural pressure is zero, the thorax will be at its *unstressed volume* (V_0), in which case the chest wall will recoil in neither direction (Fig. 32a). To say it another way, when the thorax is at its unstressed volume ($V = V_0$), the compliant parts of the chest wall are placed under no tension; thus $P_{PL} = 0$. If, while the muscles are still relaxed, air is removed from the thorax so that the thoracic volume is less than the unstressed volume ($V < V_0$), the compliant elements of the chest wall are placed under tension and recoil in the outward direction (indicated by the arrows, Fig. 32b). The outward recoil creates a negative pleural pressure. If volume is now added to the thorax (muscles relaxed) until the thoracic volume is greater than the unstressed volume ($V > V_0$), the compliant elements of the chest wall are again placed under tension and recoil in the inward direction (Fig. 32c). This inward recoil creates a positive pleural pressure.

The pressure-volume relationship obtained in this manner represents the compliance curve of the chest wall, and the change in volume divided by the change in pleural pressure defines the compliance of the chest wall. If the thorax were stiffer than normal (less compliant), the same volume added or removed from the thorax would create a greater change in pleural pressure. If the thorax were flabbier than normal (more compliant), the same volume change would create a smaller change in pleural pressure.

A hypothetical compliance curve of a normal chest wall is plotted in Figure 33. Figure 33b,c represents the volume-pressure relationships which would be obtained from chest walls of increased and decreased compliances, respectively. Although we considered the thorax as having no contents, the analysis would have been identical had the heart and lungs been in the thorax since thoracic contents merely represent volume. Thus if we took a deep breath (so that thoracic volume was greater than

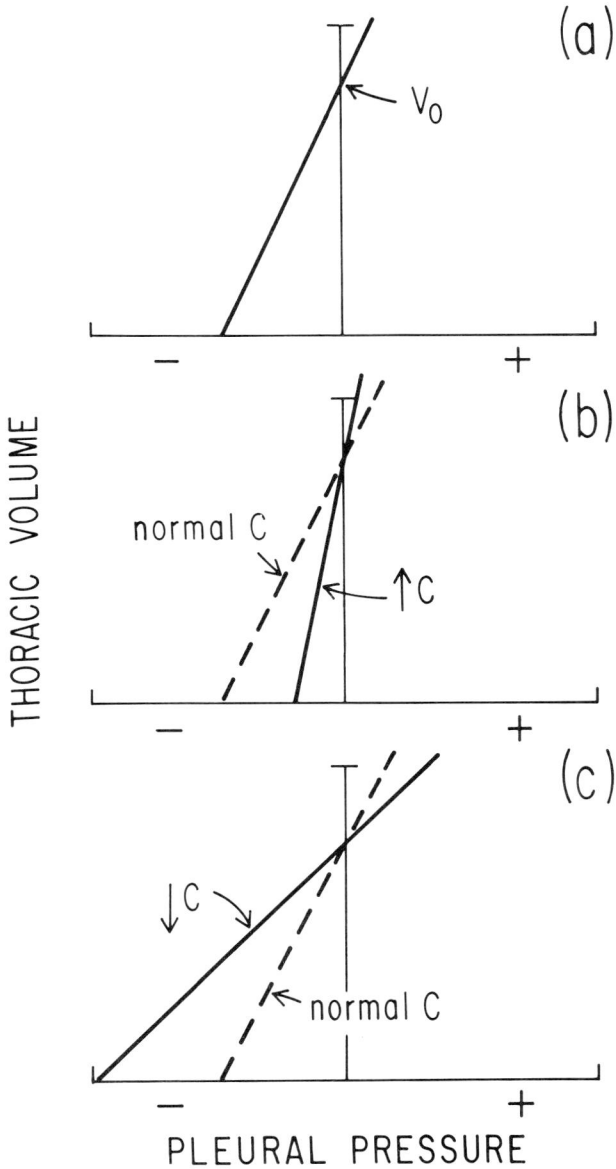

Fig. 33. a: Hypothetical pressure-volume curve of a normal chest wall. V_0=unstressed volume. b: Hypothetical pressure-volume curve of a chest wall with increased compliance, and c: with decreased compliance.

V_0) and relaxed our muscles of respiration against a closed airway, pleural pressure would become positive because of the inward recoil of the chest wall. Similarly, if we exhaled to a very low volume (so that thoracic volume was less than V_0) and relaxed our muscles of respiration against a closed airway, pleural pressure would become negative because of the outward recoil of the chest wall. Try it, and feel the direction the chest wall wants to move.

In the above example the respiratory muscles were considered relaxed. This is essential for the analysis because if the muscles were contracted (against a closed glottis) pressure swings would be superimposed on the purely elastic pressure-volume relationship. Consider what would happen at any given but constant thoracic volume. Contraction of the expiratory muscles would cause an increase in pleural pressure, whereas contraction of the inspiratory muscles would cause a decrease in the pleural pressure. The magnitude of the change in pleural pressure caused by contraction of the respiratory muscles at constant volume is related to the contractile properties of the muscles but provides no information about the elastic properties of the lung or chest wall.

In summary, the ratio of the change in lung volume to change in transthoracic pressure under conditions of relaxed respiratory muscles is by definition the compliance of the chest wall and is an index of chest wall elasticity. An important fact arising from this relationship is that the pleural pressure under relaxed conditions with glottis closed is determined only by the elastic properties of the chest wall and the volume of the thorax. If the respiratory muscles are contracted, at constant volume, the pleural pressure is further determined by the magnitude of contraction, more positive (less negative) if the expiratory muscles are contracted and less positive (more negative) if the inspiratory muscles are contracted. The presence (or absence) of the heart and lung has no effect on pleural pressure except that the volume of the thorax is usually determined by the volume of the lungs.

FUNCTIONAL RESIDUAL CAPACITY

At the end of a normal expiration, when the muscles of respiration are relaxed, the lung-chest wall system comes to rest at a volume known as the functional residual capacity (FRC). What determines FRC? The lung, although anatomically independent of the chest wall, is functionally linked to it by a thin layer of fluid which lines the visceral and parietal pleuras. This thin layer of pleural fluid actually holds the visceral and parietal pleuras together in much the same way that a thin layer of water between two sheets of glass holds the sheets together. Thus, the elastic recoil characteristics of the lung can influence the chest wall and vice versa. FRC is determined when the inward-acting recoil of the lung just balances the outward-acting recoil of the chest wall (Fig. 34). The pressure-volume curves of both the lung and the chest wall are plotted on the same coordinates in Figure 35. FRC occurs when the transmural pressure of the lungs (the

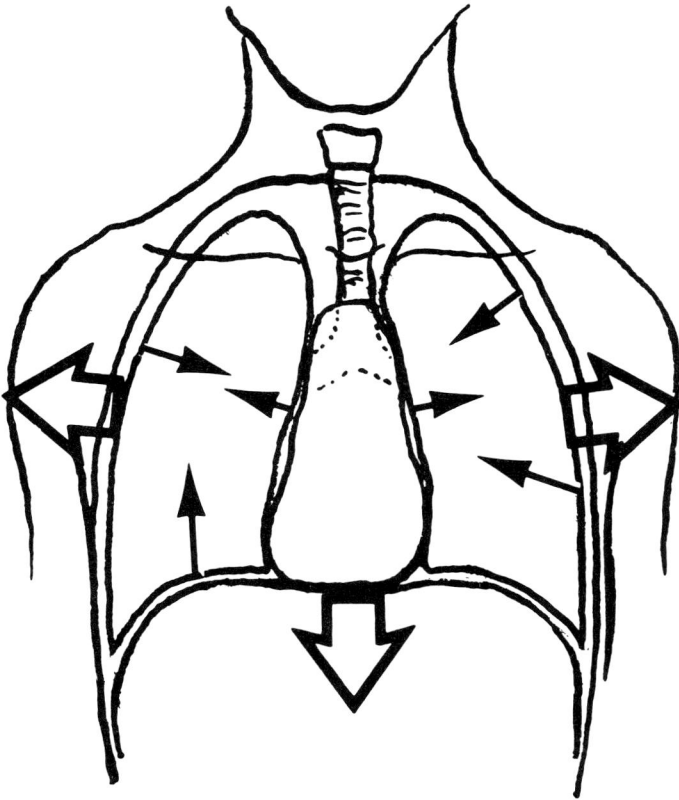

Fig. 34. Lung-chest wall system illustrated at functional residual capacity (FRC). The elastic recoil of the lung tends to pull the chest wall in and the elastic recoil of the chest wall tends to pull the lung out. FRC occurs when the inward elastic recoil of the lung just balances the outward elastic recoil of the chest wall.

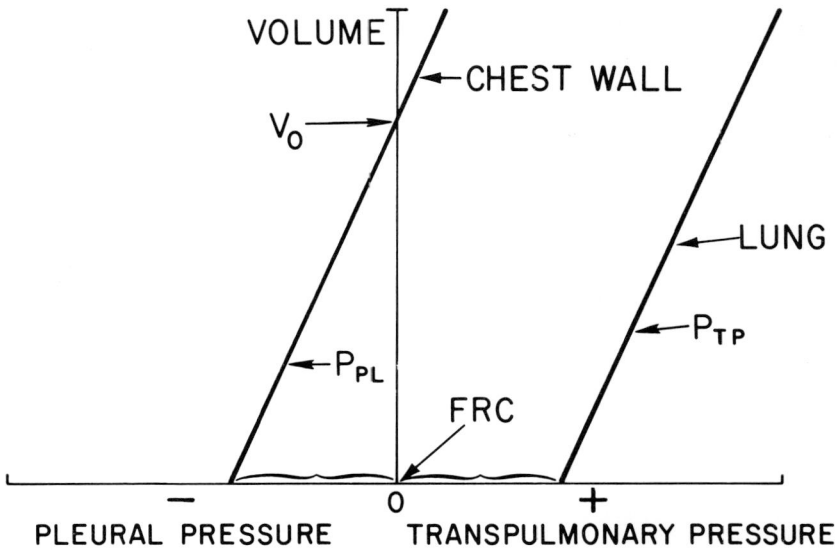

Fig. 35.   Pressure-volume curves of the lung and chest wall illustrating the determinants of functional residual capacity (FRC). FRC occurs when the elastic
recoil of the lung is equal but opposite to that of the chest wall. These
lines represent relaxation curves. They are applicable only to relaxed
expiration from TLC to FRC point. The actual pleural pressure is different
from this during normal inspiration. P_{TP}=transpulmonary pressure and
P_{PL}=pleural pressure.

transpulmonary pressure) is equal but opposite to the transmural pressure of the chest wall (the pleural pressure).

COMPLIANCE OF THE LUNG PLUS CHEST WALL

The relationship of thoracic volume to distending pressure of
the lung-chest wall system, known as the *transthoracic pressure,*
is the total compliance of the lungs plus chest wall. The transthoracic pressure (P_{TT}) is the sum of the transpulmonary pressure plus the distending pressure of the chest wall

$$P_{TT} = P_{TP} + P_{CW}$$

or

$$P_{TT} = (P_A - P_{PL}) + (P_{PL} - P_{ATM}) .$$

Since all pressures are referred to atmospheric pressure and since these measurements are usually made under static conditions, where alveolar pressure is equal to tracheal pressure (P_T)

$$P_{TT} = P_T. \qquad (23)$$

Thus, under static conditions, when the muscles of respiration are relaxed (or paralyzed) a pressure applied to the trachea opposes the elastic recoil of the lung plus the elastic recoil of the chest wall. The lung always recoils in an inward direction; however, the direction of the chest wall recoil depends upon the thoracic (lung) volume. When the thorax is at its unstressed volume (V_0) the chest wall recoils in neither direction and a pressure applied at the trachea at this volume opposes only lung recoil. It is, therefore. equal to the transpulmonary pressure.

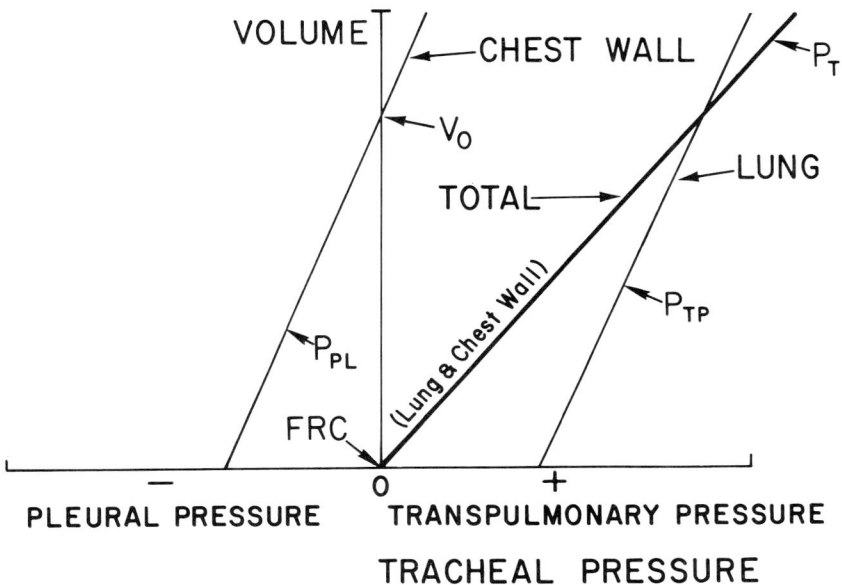

Fig. 36.   Compliance curves of the lung and chest wall and the series compliance curve (marked total) of the lung plus chest wall. P_T = tracheal pressure, P_{TP} = transpulmonary pressure, and P_{PL} = pleural pressure.

When the thorax is at a volume greater than V_0, both the lung and chest wall recoil inward, and a pressure applied at the trachea at this volume opposes the inward recoil of both the lung and chest wall. When the thorax is at a volume less than V_0, the chest wall recoil is opposite to that of the lung, and a pressure applied to the trachea at this volume is less than the transpulmonary pressure because of the "help" provided by the outward-recoiling chest wall. At FRC, when the inward recoil of the lung is just balanced by the outward recoil of the chest wall, no pressure need be applied at the trachea to oppose the elastic recoil of the lung plus chest wall. Plotted in Figure 36 are the compliant curves of the lung and chest wall, plus the series compliance curve (marked total) of the lung plus chest wall. The total curve represents the force that must be applied at the trachea to oppose the elastic recoil of the lung plus chest wall.

In summary, total distending pressure of the thorax at any volume measured at the trachea, under static conditions, is simply the sum of the transpulmonary pressure plus the recoil pressure of the chest wall and is called the transthoracic pressure. The ratio of the change in thoracic volume to change in transthoracic pressure, under static conditions, is by definition the total compliance of the thorax.

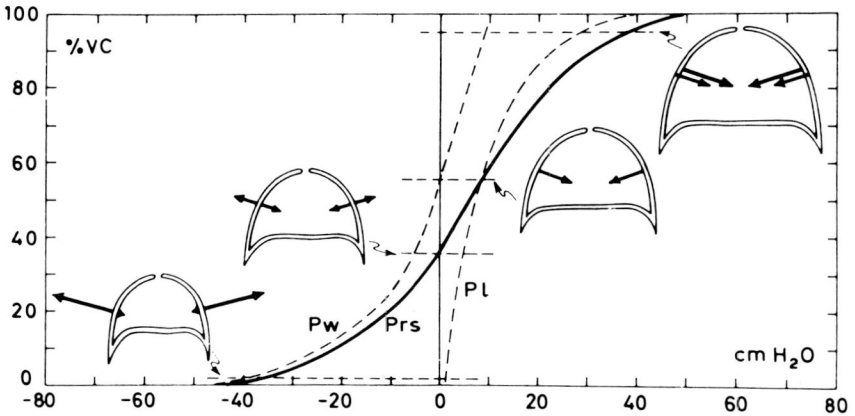

Fig. 37.   Static pressure-volume curves of the lung, chest wall, and total respiratory system during relaxation in the upright posture. The static forces of the lung and chest wall are pictured by the arrows in the drawings. The volume corresponding to each drawing is indicated by the horizontal broken lines. (From Agnostoni and Mead.[1] Reproduced with permission of *The Handbook of Physiology.*)

Until now we have assumed linear static compliance for the lung, chest wall, and total respiratory system. This assumption is correct over the middle range of lung volume, immediately above FRC; however, these compliances become alinear at high and low lung volumes. The static pressure-volume curves of the lung, chest wall, and total respiratory system over the entire range of vital capacity are presented in Figure 37.

11

Pressure-flow Relationships of the Pulmonary Airways

SPONTANEOUS VENTILATION

The pressure-flow relationships of the pulmonary airways are not unlike those of the circulatory system. Not only must the pressures and resistances be considered, but the pressure-volume relationships of the lung must also be taken into account. This is because the elasticity of the lung is in large part responsible for the driving pressure for air flow in much the same way that the elasticity of the systemic veins determines to a large extent the upstream driving pressure for venous return.

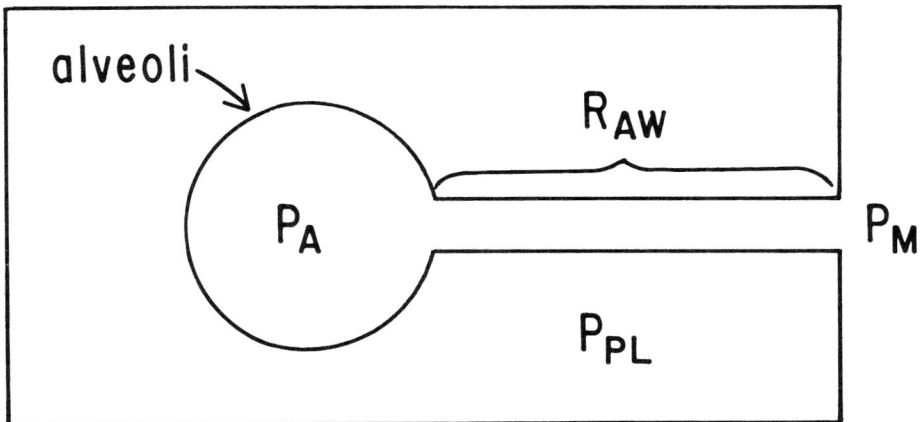

Fig. 38. Lumped parameter model of the pulmonary airways. P_A = alveolar pressure, P_M = mouth pressure, P_{PL} = pleural pressure, and R_{AW} = airway resistance.

95

A basic schematic drawing of the pulmonary airways is presented in Figure 38. This is another lumped parameter model. All alveoli are lumped together and represented by a spherical elastic element. Similarly, all airways between the mouth and the alveoli are lumped into a single equivalent airway. The box surrounding the lung represents the thorax.

There is one major difference in the pressure-flow relationships of the pulmonary airways compared with those of the circulation. In the circulation the direction of flow is always the same, i.e. from arteries to veins. In the pulmonary airway the direction of flow reverses periodically. Air moves in and out, in and out, etc. This necessitates breaking our discussion of air flow in the lungs into two categories: inspiration and expiration.

The pressure-flow relationships of the pulmonary airways during inspiration may be described by the following expression

$$\dot{V}_I = \frac{P_M - P_A}{R_{AW}}, \qquad (24)$$

where $\dot{V}_I$ = inspiratory flow,* P_M = the pressure at the mouth, P_A = pressure in the alveoli, and R_{AW} = airway resistance. The pressure-flow relationships of the pulmonary airways during expiration is similarly described by

$$\dot{V}_E = \frac{P_A - P_M}{R_{AW}}, \qquad (25)$$

where $\dot{V}_E$ = expiratory air flow. For air to be drawn into the lungs, the mouth pressure (upstream pressure) must be greater than alveolar pressure (downstream pressure). For air to be expired from the lungs, alveolar pressure (now the upstream pressure) must be greater than the downstream mouth pressure. The pressure at the mouth is, except during periods of positive pressure ventilation (see below), atmospheric pressure, and remains constant over any given respiratory cycle. Therefore, the

---

*When speaking of air, the symbol V is used to represent air volume and $\dot{V}$ to represent air volume per unit time or air flow. The symbolic language used in cardiovascular and pulmonary physiology is summarized and defined in Appendix 2.

determinants of alveolar pressure become important, for they essentially determine the magnitude of the pressure drop down the airways.

To consider alveolar pressure we must consider the pressure-volume characteristics of the lungs, a subject previously discussed in Chapter 10 in terms of pulmonary compliance. At FRC (functional residual capacity) the elastic recoil of the lung is equal and opposite to that of the chest wall, and the lung-chest wall system is stationary. Being stationary the alveolar pressure is equal to mouth pressure, there is no pressure gradient, and, therefore, no flow. The lungs nevertheless are inflated, which necessitates a positive transpulmonary pressure. This is accomplished by the subatmospheric pleural pressure which is generated by the outward recoil of the chest wall. As inspiration commences the muscles of inspiration contract, causing pleural pressure to fall. The drop in pleural pressure is transmitted to the alveoli, and alveolar pressure falls relative to mouth pres-

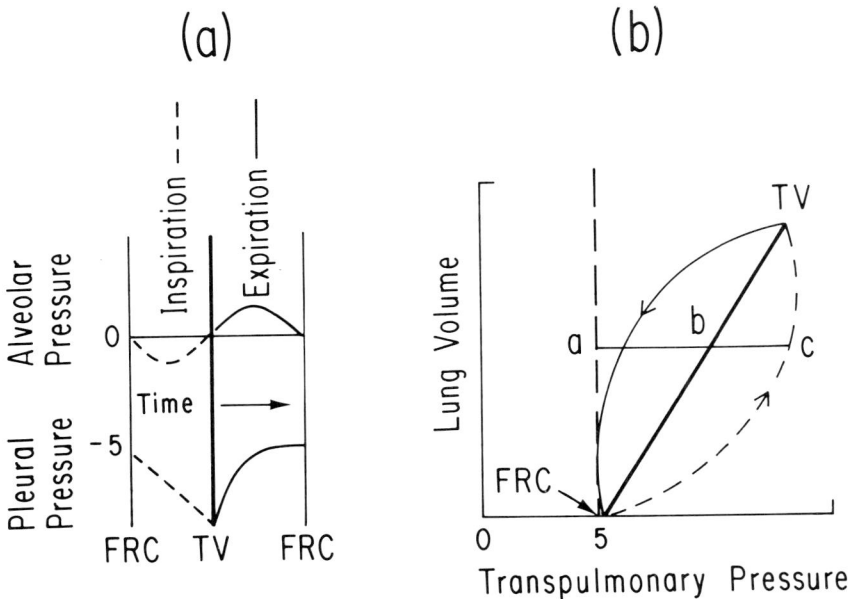

Fig. 39.   a: Respiratory pressures as a function of time throughout the respiratory cycle. FRC=functional residual capacity and TV=tidal volume. b: Pressure-volume diagram of the lung illustrating the difference between the static and dynamic transpulmonary pressure. Line segment a-b represents the static component of transpulmonary pressure, while line segment b-c represents the dynamic component.

sure.* Figure 39*a* illustrates the temporal changes in pleural and alveolar pressures which occur during inspiration and expiration.

The drop in alveolar pressure with inspiration establishes a pressure gradient and air rushes in to expand the lungs. At end-inspiration (TV, Fig. 39) the lung volume is greater than it was at FRC, and, therefore, the elastic recoil of the lung is greater. (The increase in lung volume during a normal inspiration is called a tidal volume, TV.) As the muscles of inspiration relax, the lung is allowed to recoil inward. This inward recoil is at this higher lung volume unopposed by the chest wall; therefore, the inward recoil elevates alveolar pressure relative to mouth pressure, establishing a pressure gradient for expiration. Expiration continues until the elastic recoil of the lung directed inward is once again equal to the outward recoil of the chest wall. When this occurs the lung-chest wall system has returned to FRC, alveolar pressure is equal to mouth pressure, and expiration has ended (FRC, Fig. 39).

During inspiration the dynamic transpulmonary pressure (i.e. the transpulmonary pressure measured during the period when air rushes in) increases. There are basically two components to this increase: (1) the increase in transpulmonary pressure necessary to overcome the elastic properties of the lung, the so-called static transpulmonary pressure, and (2) the further increase in dynamic transpulmonary pressure needed to overcome resistance forces, mostly resistance to air flow.

Figure 39 illustrates a hypothetical pressure-volume diagram of the lung. Initially the lung is at FRC with a transmural pressure about 5 cm H_2O. The transpulmonary pressure is then increased to 10 cm H_2O, and the lung inflates to TV. Therefore line segment FRC-TV represents the static compliance curve of the lung (Chap. 10). At any volume between the two static points the dynamic transpulmonary pressure will be greater than the static transpulmonary pressure by an amount proportional to the amount of air moving into the lung per unit time (the air flow) and the resistance to air flow. In Figure 39 line segment a–b represents the static transpulmonary pressure, line segment b–c the added component necessary to overcome the resistance to air

---

*All pressures are measured relative to atmospheric pressure. Since mouth pressure is equal to atmospheric pressure, alveolar pressure falls to a subatmospheric pressure.

flow.* From Equation 24 we can see that segment b–c would be equal to $\dot{V}_I R_{AW}$ or to alveolar pressure (mouth pressure remaining at atmospheric pressure). In a similar manner, during expiration the dynamic transpulmonary pressure will be less than the static transpulmonary pressure by an amount proportional to the air flow and the resistance to air flow.

FORCED EXPIRATION

During spontaneous breathing expiration is passive, resulting from the elastic recoil of the lung. During a forced expiration the muscles of expiration are brought into play, and the expiration becomes active. Recall that, at any given lung volume, the transpulmonary pressure is a function of the elastic property of the lungs. Thus the transpulmonary pressure can be thought of as an elastic recoil pressure, P_{EL}, such that $P_{EL} = P_A - P_{PL}$, where P_A and P_{PL} are alveolar and pleural pressures, respectively. This expression can be rearranged as

$$P_A = P_{EL} + P_{PL} . \qquad (26)$$

During a forced expiration the contraction of the expiratory muscles causes the pleural pressure to rise to a positive pressure. We can see from Equation 26 that this pressure will be transmitted directly to the alveoli. The large rise in alveolar pressure that results during an active respiratory effort produces tremendous expiratory flow. This flow, however, becomes limited at some point and greater expiratory efforts produce no increase in flow. This maximum expiratory flow ($\dot{V}_{E\,max}$) that is effort independent can be accounted for on the basis of the pressure-flow relationship of Starling resistors. The pleural pressure is the effective surrounding pressure of the large extrapulmonary intrathoracic airways. As pleural pressure rises with increasing expiratory

---

*A very small component of segment b-c would be elastic resistance created by movement or distortions of lung tissue and chest wall. Fortunately this is small enough normally to be ignored. Another component of segment b-c which at times can be significant would be pressure drops in the airways due to convection acceleration as defined by the Bernoulli equation: $P_{TP} = \dfrac{\rho}{2} \left(\dfrac{1}{A_2^2} - \dfrac{1}{A_1^2} \right) \dot{V}_I$,

where ρ = density of the air and A = area of the airway at two different points.

effort, a point is reached where it equals the pressure within these large airways. When this occurs the airways collapse and begin to function as Starling resistors. Recall (Chap. 2) that the driving pressure for flow through a Starling resistor is the upstream pressure (in this case the alveolar pressure) minus the surrounding pressure (here the pleural pressure). Applying the pressure-flow relationships of a Starling resistor to the pulmonary airway

$$\dot{V}_{E_{MAX}} = \frac{P_A - P_{PL}}{R_{AW}}. \qquad (27)$$

Substituting Equation 26 into this expression yields

$$\dot{V}_{E_{MAX}} = \frac{P_{EL}}{R_{AW}}. \qquad (28)$$

Thus, under conditions of large airway collapse the pleural pressure acts both as part of the upstream pressure (P_A) and as back pressure. The net effect is that once collapse occurs the driving pressure for flow is generated simply from the inward elastic recoil of the lung. A greater muscular effort which increases pleural pressure has no effect on flow because the effect pleural pressure has on alveolar pressure is exactly counterbalanced by the back-pressure effect of pleural pressure. A convenient way of demonstrating maximum effort-independent flow due to airway collapse is with the *expiratory volume-flow curve*.*

Figure 40 shows a series of expiratory volume-flow curves obtained from a normal healthy individual. In traces A, B, and C expiration starts at total lung capacity (TLC). Trace A shows the flow with decreasing volume to FRC during a relaxed expiration, and trace B shows the volume-flow changes during some sub-

---

*From convention, volume is plotted on the ordinate and flow on the abscissa.

maximal expiratory effort to residual volume (RV). Trace C is a maximal expiratory flow curve. Increasing the expiratory effort from TLC will not increase the flow and move the curve farther to the right of trace C, nor will any expiratory effort at any other lung volume increase the maximum expiratory flow. Trace D shows the expiratory flow during a forced expiration starting at 75 per cent TLC. Note the flow follows the maximal expiratory flow curve (trace C). If a maximal expiratory effort is started at any lung volume, the maximal flow will never exceed that of trace C, but rather it will follow C to RV. Airway collapse occurs along the descending portion of curve C. The reasons for the decreasing flow once collapse occurs is that the lung volume is decreasing as expiration continues. A lower lung volume means a lower elastic recoil (P_{EL}) and, therefore, from Equation 28, a lower flow. Thus, Equation 28 can represent an infinite number of points along the descending limb of the expiratory volume-flow curve depending upon lung volume, which is constantly changing.

Another way of looking at effort-independent expiratory flow caused by large airway collapse is through the *isovolume pressure-flow relationship*. If at any volume in Figure 40 a horizontal line is drawn it can be seen that flow will increase with increasing effort (we go from trace A to trace B to trace C); thereafter flow will show no further increase despite increasing effort (there is no curve to the right of C). Expiratory effort may be measured as the difference between the pressure within the alveoli (P_A) and mouth pressure (P_M), ΔP. Figure 41 illustrates schematically the airway dynamics which are responsible for the isovolume pressure-flow curve. Figure 42 shows a series of isovolume pressure-flow curves obtained in the human at different lung volumes. The expiratory air flow of the human subject was interrupted at a selected lung volume; the subject then increased expiratory effort against a closed valve until the mouth pressure (which was equal to alveolar pressure since flow was zero) reached a preset value at which the valve opened. Expiratory flow immediately after the valve opened was plotted against mouth pressure (alveolar pressure) immediately before valve opening. This procedure was repeated multiple times at the same lung volume, then at different lung volumes. Thus, each curve presented in Figure 42 was constructed from multiple data points. Note that flow increased as effort increased until a critical ΔP was reached; thereafter flow remained relatively constant (trace C in Fig. 40 had been reached). At the critical ΔP where flow remained constant the airways collapsed.

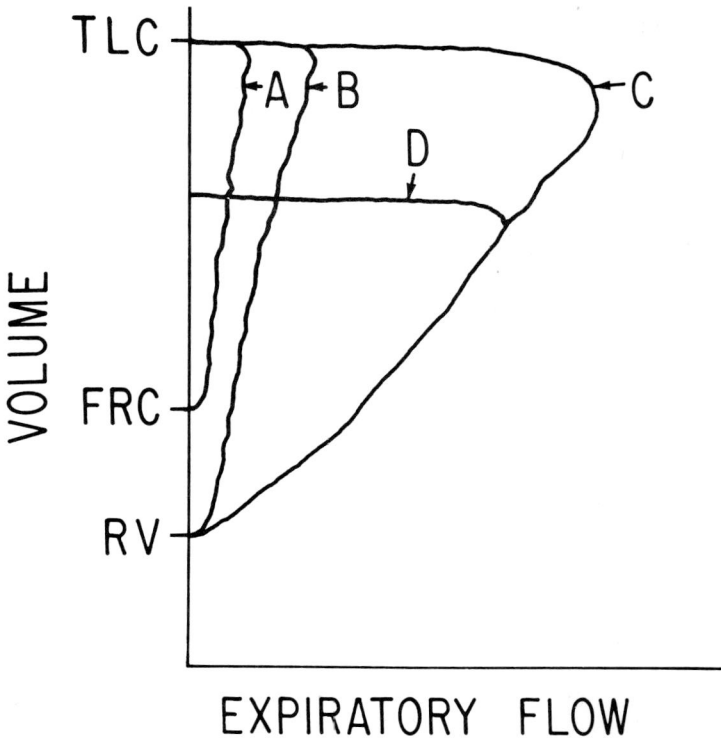

Fig. 40. Expiratory volume-flow curves. TLC = total lung capacity, FRC = functional residual capacity, and RV = residual volume.

Fig. 41. Schematic drawing of the airway dynamics responsible for the isovolume pressure-flow curve. The collapsible portion of the airway is represented in the model by wavy lines. Panel a illustrates a static condition. Pleural pressure is −5 units, and alveolar pressure is atmospheric. Since the pressure drop down the airways is zero, flow is zero. Transpulmonary pressure is 5 units and will remain 5 in all panels since the lung volume will remain the same (isovolume). As expiratory effort is begun (panel b) and pleural pressure rises from −5 to 0 to +1 (panel c), alveolar pressure rises from 0 to +5 to +6. As a pressure gradient between alveoli and mouth (ΔP) is now established, flow begins and increases. As flow increases the equal pressure point (EPP) or the point where airway pressure equals pleural pressure moves back toward the alveoli. In panel d pleural pressure has risen sufficiently to cause the equal pressure point to reach the collapsible segment of airway. When this occurs the airway collapses and begins to function as a Starling resistor, i.e. the pleural pressure becomes the back pressure. Once collapse occurs any further rise in pleural pressure (panels e and f) results in an equal rise in alveolar pressure and back pressure; therefore, the pressure gradient for flow $(P_a - P_{PE})$ remains constant and flow remains constant despite an increasing ΔP $(P_A - P_M)$.

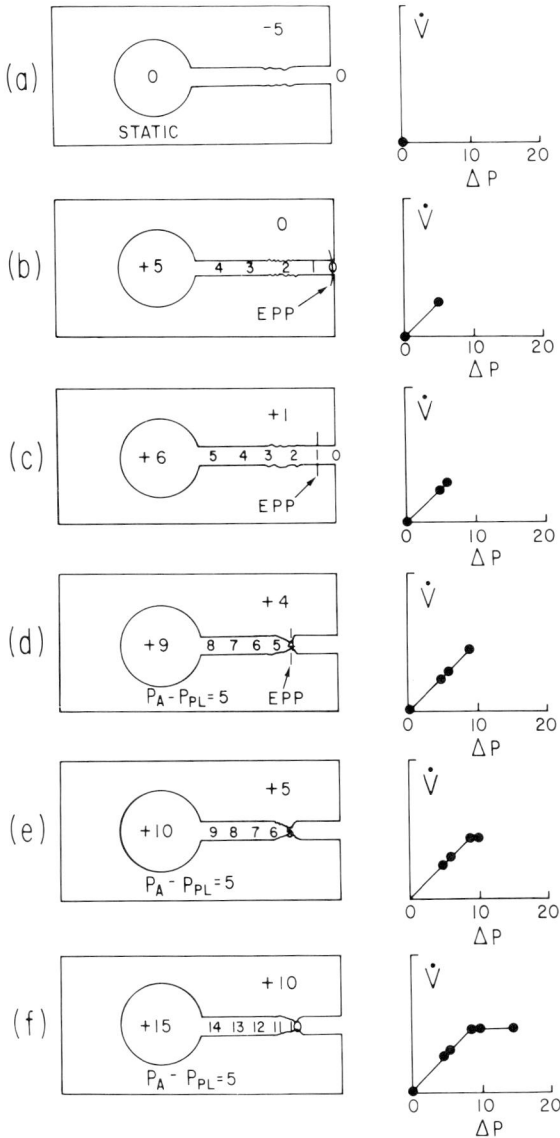

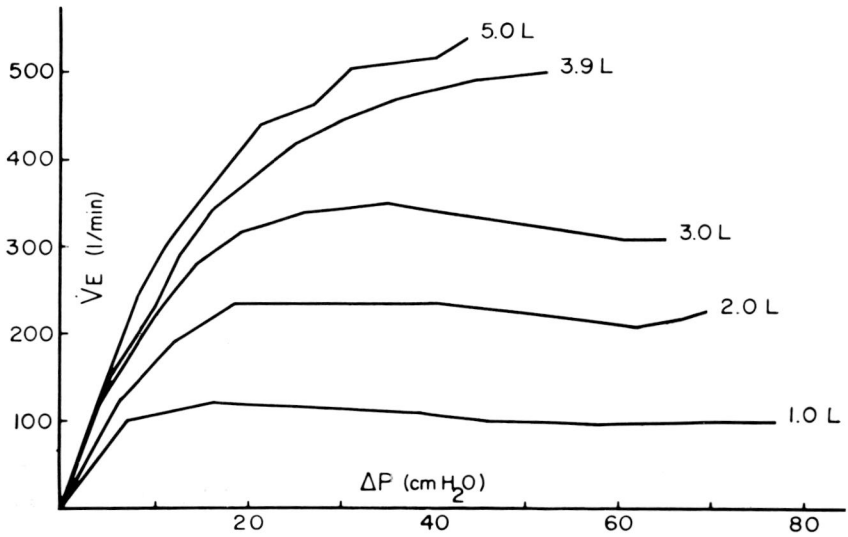

Fig. 42. A family of isovolume pressure-flow curves at different lung volumes above residual volume in a normal man. Note that the greater the lung volume, the greater is the flow when airway collapse occurs (plateau). Contrast these isovolume pressure-flow curves with the expiratory volume-flow curve presented in Figure 40. (From Pride et al.[32] Reproduced with permission of the American Physiological Society.)

In Chapter 2 we discussed the pressure-flow relationships of collapsible tubes and presented a plot of flow against the difference between inflow and outflow pressures for a hypothetical example (Fig. 8a). A comparison of Figure 42 with Figure 8 will reveal marked similarities. They are similar because they represent the same phenomenon.

12

Practical Aspects of Pulmonary Mechanics

Respiratory disorders are numerous and complex. It is not the purpose of this chapter to characterize each respiratory dysfunction. For this the student is referred to several excellent monographs.[4,10] Two major categories of respiratory dysfunction are primarily related to alterations in the mechanical properties of the lung. In this chapter our discussion will demonstrate how the knowledge of normal pulmonary mechanics can serve as a basis for the conceptual understanding of the pathophysiology (altered mechanics) of these two major categories of pulmonary disease.

Pulmonary dysfunctions resulting from abnormalities of the mechanical properties of the lungs include those which result from alteration in the pressure-volume relation, the *restrictive diseases*, and those which result from alterations in the pressure-flow relationship, the *obstructive diseases*.

ABNORMAL PRESSURE-VOLUME RELATIONSHIPS OF THE LUNG AND CHEST WALL

The elastic properties of the lung are defined in terms of the static pulmonary compliance: the ratio of the change in lung volume to change in transpulmonary pressure under static conditions.* If the lungs are stiffer than normal, the ratio will be

---

*The dynamic compliance (C_{dyn}) is another measure of lung elasticity. It is simply the compliance measured during the respiratory cycle. Unfortunately the dynamic compliance does not always equal the static compliance. This is because airway obstruction in one region of the lung will cause that region to fill with air more slowly than other regions. Less air will, therefore, go into that region. The faster the breathing frequency, the less will be the ΔV for that region. Thus, with airway obstruction, C_{dyn} becomes frequency dependent and decreases as the breathing frequency increases. For this reason C_{dyn} must be interpreted with caution.

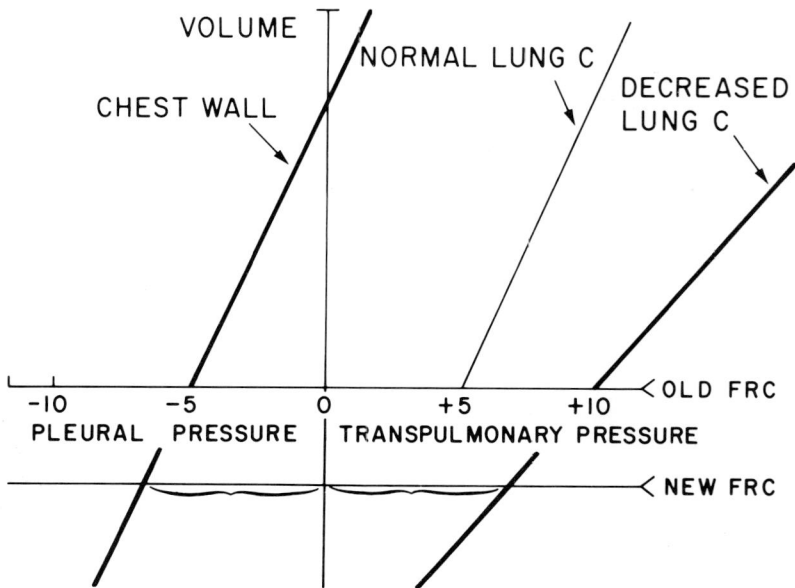

Fig. 43. Pressure-volume relationships of a hypothetical stiff lung. The chest wall and normal lung compliance curves are identical to those presented in Fig. 35. Decreasing lung compliance reduces FRC and increases the transpulmonary pressure necessary to inflate the lung to any given volume.

smaller than normal; if the lungs are flabbier than normal, the ratio will be larger than normal. An important characteristic of a stiff lung is a restriction in the ability of the lung to fully expand. Thus, this type of condition is often called a restrictive disease. Examples of restrictive diseases include diffuse interstitial fibrosis, pulmonary edema, and pulmonary scleroderma. The chief characteristic of a flabby lung is an overdistension of the lung. The classical example of this disease state is emphysema.

Figure 43 presents the pressure-volume relationship of a hypothetical stiff lung. The decreased compliance necessitates a higher-than-normal transpulmonary pressure to inflate the lung to any given volume. The FRC is lowered by the decreased lung compliance, because the increased lung recoil pulls the chest wall in until the outward recoil of the chest wall becomes equal but opposite to the inward recoil of the lung.

Figure 44 presents the pressure-volume relationship of a hypothetical flabby lung. The increased lung compliance allows a much greater lung volume at any given transpulmonary pres-

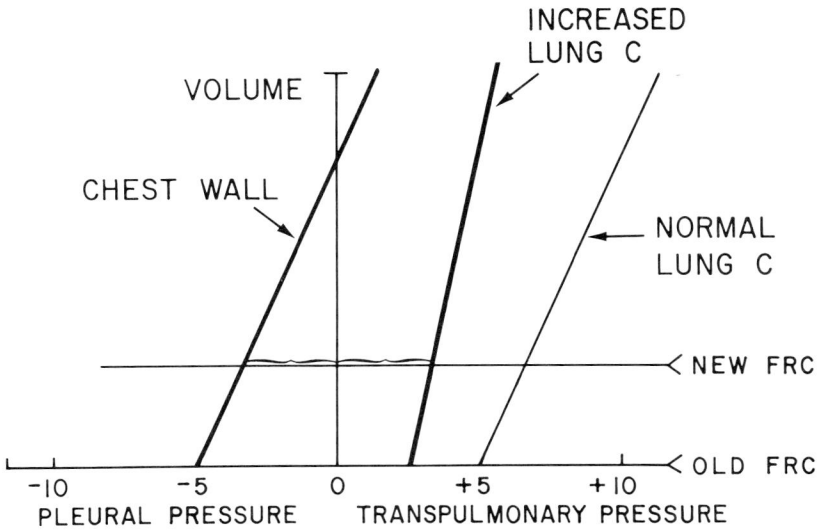

Fig. 44. Pressure-volume relationships of a hypothetical flabby lung. Increasing lung compliance increases FRC and reduces the transpulmonary pressure necessary to inflate the lung to any given volume.

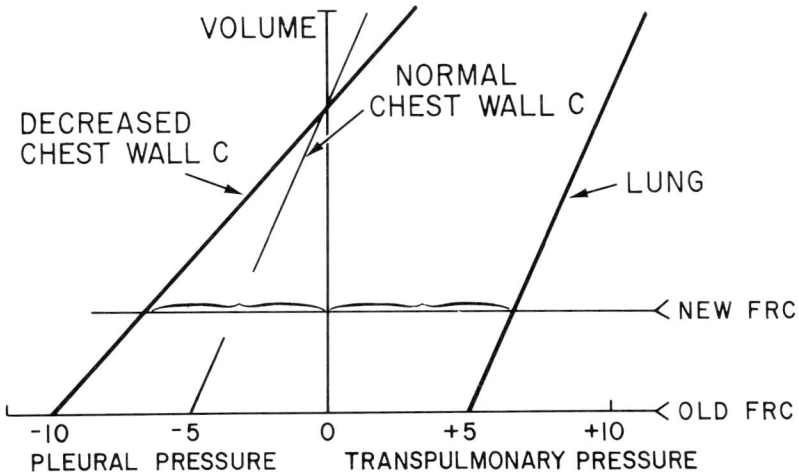

Fig. 45. Pressure-volume relationships of a hypothetical stiff chest wall. The decreased chest wall compliance increases FRC and increases the amount of work the patient must do to ventilate normally.

sure. Note that reducing the elastic recoil of the lung increases FRC. The inward recoil of the more compliant lung is only to balance the outward recoil of the normal chest wall at a higher-than-normal lung volume.

A restrictive disease of the chest wall, such as kyphoscoliosis, will also increase FRC. Figure 45 illustrates in another hypothetical example how this will occur. The increased outward recoil of the chest wall because of its decreased compliance actually pulls the lung out to a higher volume. The inward recoil of the lung is then equal but opposite to the outward recoil of the chest wall. There is no known disease which increases the compliance of the chest wall.

ABNORMAL PRESSURE-FLOW AND VOLUME-FLOW RELATIONSHIPS OF THE LUNG

Recall from Chapter 11 that during a forced expiration the expiratory flow ($\dot{V}_E$) is determined by the magnitude of the alveolar pressure and the total airway resistance between alveoli and mouth (Eq. 25). Once the airways collapse a maximum effort-independent flow is achieved which is determined by the magnitude of the elastic recoil of the lung and the airway resistance up to the collapsed portion of the airway (Eq. 28). Collapse normally occurs at very high flows and pressures and in relatively large airways (0.3 mm in diameter) which possess bronchial smooth muscle. Under some conditions (reversible obstructive airway disease), this bronchial smooth muscle will contract and result in collapse of the large airways at lower than normal intrapleural pressures. Pride et al.[32] have used this fact, together with the special characteristics of Starling resistors (Chaps. 2 and 6), to account for the difference between reversible and irreversible obstructive airway disease. Their analysis provides a useful conceptual basis for the understanding of the pathophysiology of these conditions. They assumed that under normal conditions, when the bronchial smooth muscle tone is zero (or the bronchial wall has sufficient stiffness to counteract the tone), the pleural pressure (P_{PL}) is the effective back pressure to air flow from the lung, as described by Equation 27. As bronchial smooth muscle tone increases it generates an inward-acting pressure which augments the pleural pressure. Thus, under conditions of increased bronchial tone

$$\dot{V}_{EMAX} = \frac{P_A - P_{TM}'}{R_{AW}}, \tag{29}$$

where $P_{TM'}$ is the sum of all collapsing forces (pleural pressure plus bronchial smooth muscle tone) and R_{AW} is the resistance of the airway up to the point of collapse. On the basis of this analysis, Pride et al. postulated that reversible airway obstruction, such as asthma, results from an increase in bronchial

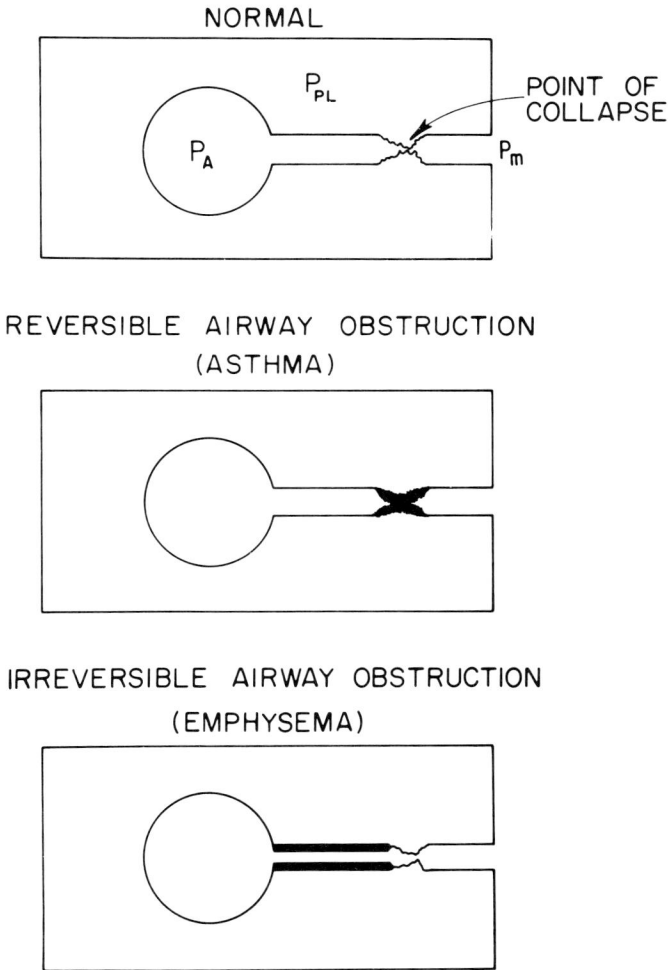

Fig. 46.   Lumped parameter model of the pulmonary airways. P_A = alveolar pressure, P_{PL} = pleural pressure, and P_M = mouth pressure. Reversible airway obstruction is characterized as an increase in the bronchiole smooth muscle tone at the point of collapse. Irreversible airways obstruction is characterized as a permanent change in the dimension of the upstream airways resistance between the alveoli and the bronchiole waterfall.

smooth muscle tone in the large collapsible airways, whereas irreversible airway obstruction, such as emphysema, is a manifestation of a permanent increase in the airway resistance in the small airways between the alveoli and the collapsible portion of the large airways. Figure 46 illustrates this difference schematically.

When analyzed in terms of an isovolume pressure-flow curve (Chap. 11), an irreversible airway disease simply reduces the initial slope of the pressure-flow curve (Fig. 47a) whereas the critical pressure difference ($\Delta P'$) where collapse occurs does not change. In contrast, reversible airway disease does not change the slope of the pressure-flow curve but reduces the $\Delta P'$ where collapse occurs (Fig. 47b). After the disease process is reversed the isovolume pressure-flow curve reverts to normal.

Asthma

Asthma is an obstructive disease which has been characterized as an increase in the collapsing force of the large airways (Fig. 46). The elastic recoil of the lung is usually normal but may be transiently decreased because the obstruction to expiratory flow increases lung volume and causes the patient to "operate" on a higher and less compliant part of the pressure-volume curve (Fig. 37). Sometimes irreversible obstruction of small airways coexists with the obstruction of large airways. This would result in a marked reduction in expiratory flow by not only a reduction in $\Delta P'$ (Fig. 47b) but also a reduction in the slope of the isovolume pressure-flow curve (Fig. 47a). If obstruction of large airways is the primary flow-limiting factor, the administration of bronchodilators will return flow to normal.

Early Chronic Obstructive Pulmonary Disease (C.O.P.D.)

Early C.O.P.D. is characterized by an irreversible increase in small airway resistance which considerably reduces expiratory flow (Fig. 47a). Following the administration of bronchodilators, flow generally increases only slightly. The pressure-volume characteristics of the lung are usually normal.

Severe Chronic Obstructive Pulmonary Disease

Severe C.O.P.D. is characterized not only by an increased small airway resistance but also by an elevated large airway resistance. Varying degrees of loss of lung recoil may be noted. Severe

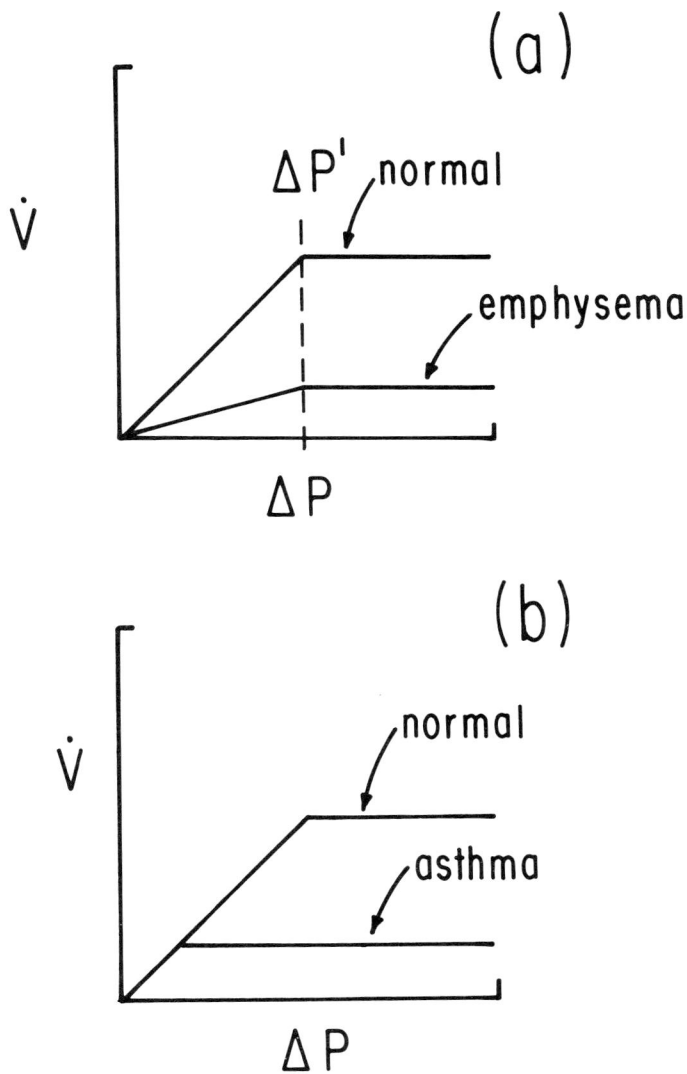

Fig. 47. Hypothetical isovolume pressure-flow curve for an irreversible airway disease (a) and a reversible airway disease (b).

flow limitation occurs and there is little or no improvement with the use of bronchodilators. Pathologically, severe C.O.P.D. is characterized by the presence of chronic bronchitis and emphysema. The former results in poorly reversible large and small airway obstruction. The pathophysiologic consequences of emphysema are summarized in the next paragraph.

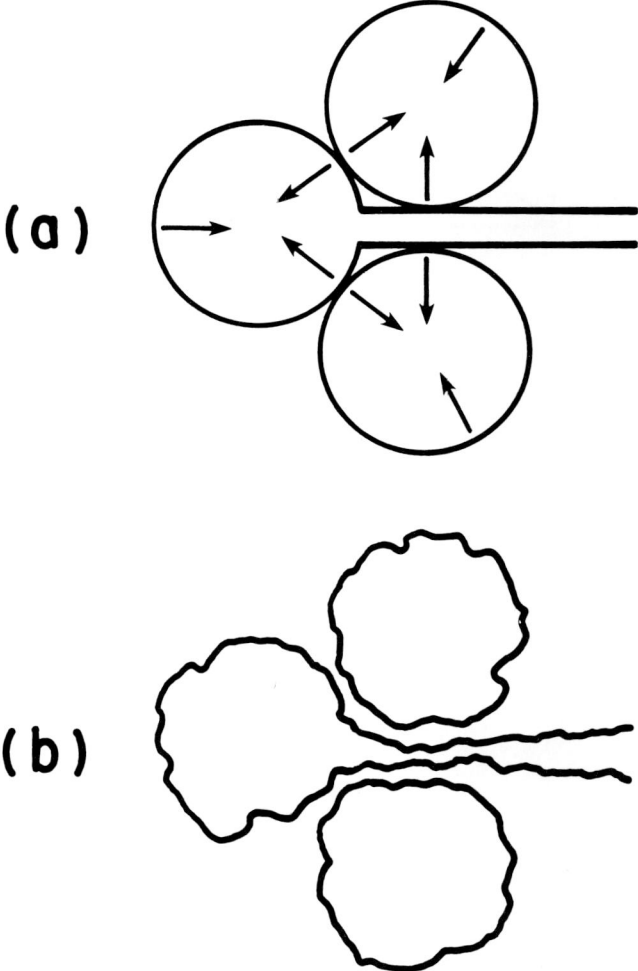

Fig. 48.　Schematic diagram illustrating the loss of elastic recoil which emphysema produces. a: A normal lung, b: An emphysemic lung.

Emphysema

Emphysema is characterized by a loss of elastic recoil. This loss not only increases lung compliance but reduces the normal radial traction that alveoli provide to small airways (Fig. 48). The loss of this radial traction causes an increased degree of small airway collapse during expiration, increasing resistance. The maximum expiratory flow is severely reduced since $P_{EL} \downarrow \downarrow / R_{AW} \uparrow$ (Eq. 28). Bronchodilators have no effect. The increased compliance of the lung also results in elevation of the FRC point and the TLC (total lung capacity, the total intrapulmonary air at the maximal inspiratory point).

SECTION IV: STUDY QUESTIONS

13

Study Questions for Section I

1. What is the gravitational force exerted by 1 ml of water?
   Solution:
   > (a) *Force* (F) is that which, acting on a *mass* (m), produces a proportionate *acceleration* (a), i.e. $F = m \cdot a$.
   >
   > (b) The unit of force in the cgs system is the *dyne*. One dyne is the force required to accelerate 1 gm 1 cm/sec^2.
   >
   > (c) The acceleration due to the earth's gravity is 980 cm/sec^2.
   >
   > (d) A mass of 1 gm exerts a force of 980 $gm \cdot cm/sec^2$ or 980 dynes.
   >
   > (e) One ml of water has a mass of 1 gm.

   Answer:
   The gravitational force exerted by 1 ml of water = 980 dynes.

2. What pressure is exerted by a column of water 1 cm^2 cross-sectional area, 1 cm in height (1 cm^3)?
   Solution:
   > (a) The gravitational force exerted by 1 cm^3 (1 ml = 1 cm^3) of water = 980 dynes.
   >
   > (b) $P = F/A = dynes/cm^2$.

   Answer:
   One cm^3 of water, 1 cm^2 cross-sectional area, exerts a pressure of 980 $dynes/cm^2$.
   Comment:
   The force *per unit area* or the pressure would be the same regardless of the total cross-sectional area. Another way of expressing the answer to this question would be the pressure equal to 1 cm H_2O or P = 1 cm H_2O.

3. What is the pressure exerted by a column of water 10 cm high?
   Solution:

   > (a) A 1-cm column of water = 980 dynes/cm².
   > (b) A 10-cm column of water = 10 times 980 dynes/cm².

   Answer:
   A 10-cm column of water equals a pressure of 9800 dynes/cm² or simply 10 cm H_2O.

4. What is the pressure exerted by a column of mercury 10 cm high?
   Solution:

   > (a) Mercury has a density 13.55 times that of water (13.55 gm/cm³).
   > (b) A column of mercury, therefore, exerts a pressure 13.55 times 980 = 13,279 dynes/cm³ for each cm height.

   Answer:
   A 10-cm column of mercury equals a pressure of 132,790 dynes/cm² or simply 10 cm mercury.
   Comment:
   Since a column of mercury exerts a pressure of 1,328 dynes/cm² for each mm in height we can convert from mm Hg pressure to dynes/cm² pressure by multiplying by 1,328. Furthermore, since 1 mm Hg = 1.355 cm H_2O we can convert a pressure measured in units of mm Hg to a pressure measured in units of cm H_2O by multiplying mm Hg by 1.355 or cm H_2O pressure into mm Hg pressure by multiplying cm H_2O by 0.738.

5. Are pressure and tension similar quantities?
   Solution:

   > (a) Pressure = F/A = dynes/cm².
   > (b) Tension = F/A = dynes/cm².

   Answer:
   Yes.

6. If pressure and tension are similar quantities, what about Young's modulus (Y) and the reciprocal of the compliance (1/C)?

Solution:
   (a) Solve Equation 1 for Y

$$Y = \frac{F \cdot L_0}{A(L - L_0)} = \frac{\text{dynes} \cdot \text{cm}}{\text{cm}^2 \cdot \text{cm}} = \text{dynes/cm}^2$$

   (b) Solve Equation 3 for 1/C

$$1/C = \frac{P}{V - V_0} = \frac{F}{A(V - V_0)} = \frac{\text{dynes}}{\text{cm}^2 \cdot \text{cm}^3} = \text{dynes/cm}^5$$

Answer:
Y and 1/C are, therefore, not similar.
Comment:
Although not strictly similar, these values nevertheless provide qualitative estimates of elasticity. Young's modulus is similar to the reciprocal of distensibility, D. Distensibility is a term used to mean the *percentage* increase in volume, thus

$$1/D = \frac{P \cdot V_0}{(V - V_0)} = \frac{F \cdot V_0}{A(V - V_0)} = \frac{\text{dynes} \cdot \text{cm}^3}{\text{cm}^2 \cdot \text{cm}^3} = \text{dynes/cm}^2$$

where V_0 = the unstressed volume. In most physiologic systems, it is not necessary to know the percentage increase in volume but only the volume increase for a given change in pressure, i.e. the compliance.

7. What are the cgs units of resistance (R)?
   Solution:
      (a) $R = P/\dot{Q}$, where P is a pressure difference, $\dot{Q}$ is a flow.
      (b) $R = 8\eta L/\pi r^4$, where η is the viscosity, L is the length of the tube, and r is the radius of the tube.
      (c) The unit for viscosity is the poise, 1 poise being equal to 1 dyne·sec/cm².

Answer:

$$\text{(a)} \ R = P/\dot{Q} = \frac{\text{dynes/cm}^2}{\text{cm}^3/\text{sec}} = \frac{\text{dynes} \cdot \text{sec}}{\text{cm}^5} =$$

$$\text{dynes} \cdot \text{sec} \cdot \text{cm}^{-5}.$$

$$\text{(b)} \ R = 8\eta L/\pi r^4 = \frac{(\text{dynes} \cdot \text{sec/cm}^2)\text{cm}}{\text{cm}^4} =$$

$$\text{dynes} \cdot \text{sec/cm}^5 = \text{dynes} \cdot \text{sec} \cdot \text{cm}^{-5}.$$

8. (A) Which factor determining resistance has the most important effect on flow?
(B) How would doubling this factor influence resistance (R)?
(C) How would doubling this factor influence flow ($\dot{Q}$)?
Solution:
$R = 8\eta L/r^4.$
Answer:
(A) The radius, r, since it is raised to the fourth power, has the most important effect on flow.
(B) Doubling r would decrease R 16 times.
(C) Doubling r would decrease $\dot{Q}$ 16 times.
Comment:
The radius is especially important in determining acute changes in resistance in the circulatory system because length and viscosity tend to remain constant over a brief period of time.

9. The pressure in the inflow reservoir (P_1) feeding a rigid water flowing system is maintained at 73.8 mm Hg. The outflow pressure is zero (atmospheric pressure). How much would the driving pressure for this system be reduced if the inflow pressure was lowered 50 cm below the point of outflow (below the horizontal)?
Solution:
    (a) Recall Equation 7: $P_{1 \text{ eff}} = P_1 - \rho gh$.
    (b) $\rho = 1.0$ gm/cm^3.
    (c) $g = 980$ cm/sec^2.
    (d) $h = 50$ cm.
    (e) $\rho gh = 49{,}000$ gm/cm$\cdot$sec$^2 = $ dynes/cm^2.
    (f) To convert to mm Hg divide by 1328.

Answer:
$P_{I\ eff}$ = 73.8 − 36.9 = 36.9 mm Hg.
Thus, the driving pressure would have been reduced by one half.
Comment:
An easier way of doing this problem would have been to convert 73.8 mm Hg into cm H_2O by multiplying by 1.355 (P_I = 100 cm H_2O), then realizing that since ρ and g are constants $\rho g h$ simply equals 50 cm H_2O. Therefore, $P_{I\ eff}$ = 100 − 50 = 50 cm H_2O, or the driving pressure was reduced by one half.

10. Water is flowing through a *rigid* tube. Let P_I = inflow pressure, P_O = outflow pressure, P_S = surrounding pressure, $\dot{Q}$ = flow, and R = resistance. Assume a constant R of 1 mm Hg·l^{-1}·min, P_I of 20 mm Hg, and P_S = 0 mm Hg. What would be the flow when
    (A) P_O = −10 mm Hg?
    (B) P_O = +5 mm Hg?
    (C) P_O = +15 mm Hg?
    Increase P_S to +10 mm Hg. What would be the flow with this new surrounding pressure when
    (D) P_O = −10 mm Hg?
    (E) P_O = +5 mm Hg?
    (F) P_O = +15 mm Hg?
    Graphical Solution (Fig. 49a):
        (a) To solve this problem graphically construct volume and pressure coordinants with volume on the ordinate and pressure on the abscissa. Starting at P = 20 mm Hg and $\dot{Q}$ = 0 l/min, plot a pressure-flow curve with a slope of −1.0 mm Hg·l^{-1}·min (Fig. 49a).
        (b) From this pressure-flow curve read the answers for Question 10 A–F.
    Mathematical Solution
        (a) Restate Poiseuille's law (Eq. 5):
$$\dot{Q} = \left(\frac{1}{R}\right) P_I - P_O$$
        (b) Substitute the appropriate values and solve for $\dot{Q}$.
    Answers:
    (A) $\dot{Q}$ = 30 l/min.
    (B) $\dot{Q}$ = 15 l/min.
    (C) $\dot{Q}$ = 5 l/min.
    (D) $\dot{Q}$ = 30 l/min.

(E) $\dot{Q}$ = 15 l/min.
(F) $\dot{Q}$ = 5 l/min.
Comment:
For a rigid system P_S does not affect the flow.

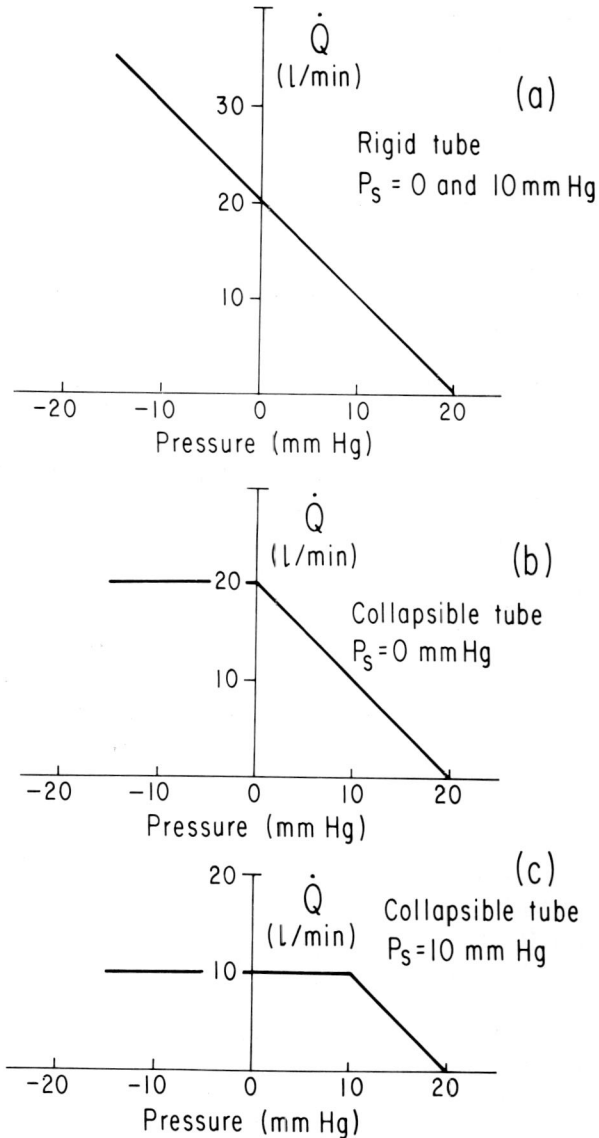

Fig. 49.   Graphic solution to Questions 10 and 11.

11. Water is flowing through a *collapsible* tube. Let P_I = inflow pressure, P_O = outflow pressure, P_S = surrounding pressure, $\dot{Q}$ = flow, R = resistance. Assume a constant R of 1 mm $Hg \cdot l^{-1} \cdot min$, P_I of 20 mm Hg, and P_S = 0 mm Hg. What would be the flow when
    (A) P_O = −10 mm Hg?
    (B) P_O = +5 mm Hg?
    (C) P_O = +15 mm Hg?
    Increase P_S to +10 mm Hg. What would be the flow with this new surrounding pressure when
    (D) P_O = −10 mm Hg?
    (E) P_O = +5 mm Hg?
    (F) P_O = +15 mm Hg?
    Graphic Solution (Fig. 49*b*, *c*):
        (a) Plot coordinates as for Question 10.
        (b) Plot two pressure-flow curves with a slope of −1.0 mm $Hg \cdot l^{-1} \cdot min$, one between pressures of 0.0 and 20 mm Hg (Fig. 49*b*) and the other between pressures of 10 and 20 mm Hg (Fig. 49*c*).
        (c) Recall that in a collapsible system whenever $P_S \geq P_O$, $\dot{Q}$ becomes independent of P_O.
        (d) For pressures less than P_S maintain flow constant.
        (e) From the appropriate pressure-flow curves read the answers for Question 11 A–F.
    Mathematical Solution:
        (a) Restate Poiseuille's law for rigid tubes (Eq. 5):

$$\dot{Q} = \frac{1}{R} (P_I - P_O)$$

        (b) Restate Poiseuille's law modified for collapsible tubes (Eq. 6):

$$\dot{Q} = \frac{1}{R} (P_I - P_S)$$

        (c) Recall that whenever $P_S < P_O$ a collapsible tube functions as a rigid tube; therefore, substitute the appropriate values into Equation 5 for conditions where $P_S < P_O$ and solve for $\dot{Q}$.
        (d) Recall that whenever $P_S \geq P_O$, P_S becomes the effective back pressure for a collapsible tube; therefore, substitute the appropriate values into Equation 6 for conditions where $P_S \geq P_O$ and solve for $\dot{Q}$.

Answers:
(A) $\dot{Q}$ = 20 l/min.
(B) $\dot{Q}$ = 15 l/min.
(C) $\dot{Q}$ = 5 l/min.
(D) $\dot{Q}$ = 10 l/min.
(E) $\dot{Q}$ = 10 l/min.
(F) $\dot{Q}$ = 5 l/min.
Comment:
For a collapsible system whenever $P_s \geq P_o$, P_o does not affect flow.

14

Study Questions for Section II

Assume for the following questions that the systemic arterial and venous compliances for man are 0.067 and 2.570 ml · kg^{-1} · mm Hg^{-1}, respectively.

12. How much blood volume would have to be injected into the systemic venous system of a 70-kg man to raise the mean systemic pressure (P_{MS}) 5 mm Hg?

    Solution:

    (a) Recall that the ratio of the change in volume to the change in pressure is the compliance of the system.

    (b) For the systemic venous system $C_V = \Delta V/\Delta P_{MS}$, where C_V = systemic venous compliance (2.570 ml · kg^{-1} · mm Hg^{-1}), ΔV = the change in blood volume.

    (c) Solving this expression for ΔV yields
    $$\Delta V = \Delta P_{MS} \cdot C_V$$

    Answer:
    $$\Delta V = 5 \cdot 2.570 \cdot 70 = 899 \text{ ml}$$
    $$\text{ml} = \text{mm Hg} \cdot \frac{\text{(ml/kg)} \cdot \text{kg}}{\text{mm Hg}}$$

13. If this same volume were injected into the systemic arterial system of a 70-kg man, what would be the change in pressure?

    Solution:

    (a) For the systemic arterial system
    $C_A = \Delta V/\Delta P_A$, where C_A = arterial compliance (0.067 ml · kg^{-1} · mm Hg^{-1}) ΔP_A = change in arterial pressure.

    (b) Solving this expression for P_A yields
    $$\Delta P_A = \Delta V/C_A$$

125

Mechanical Concepts in CVP Physiology

Answer:

$P_A = 899/(0.067 \cdot 70) = 192$ mm Hg

$$\text{mm Hg} = \frac{\text{ml}}{\frac{(\text{ml/kg})\text{kg}}{\text{mm Hg}}}$$

Comment:

It should be obvious from the above two study questions why the veins are called the capacitance vessels. The arteries cannot accommodate large quantities of blood without tremendous rises in pressure, whereas the veins are able to do this quite nicely.

14. Could this volume have come from the pulmonary circulation? Why or why not?

    Solution:

    (a) The lumped pulmonary compliance (C_P) is approximately .265 ml $\cdot$ kg^{-1} $\cdot$ mm Hg^{-1} (Table 1).

    (b) $\Delta P_{MP} = \Delta V/C_P$, where ΔP_{MP} = the change in mean pulmonary pressure, ΔV_P = the change in pulmonary blood volume.

    Answer:

    If the pulmonary system of a 70-kg man held 899 ml of blood volume (which it could release to the systemic system) its mean pulmonary pressure would be approximately 48 mm Hg, a value incompatible with life since this pressure would produce severe pulmonary edema. Therefore, it can be concluded that the pulmonary vessels do not hold the amount of volume necessary to elevate the mean systemic pressure 5 mm Hg.

    Comment:

    Because of the relatively low compliance of the pulmonary vessels the pulmonary circulation cannot be a "vascular reservoir" able to transfer volume to the systemic circulation in time of need.

15. Suppose that, for a 70-kg man, the arterial compliance (C_A) upstream from the major site of arterial resistance (R_A) was equal to the venous compliance (C_V), such that $C_A = C_V = 2.57$ ml $\cdot$ kg^{-1} $\cdot$ mm Hg^{-1}. Let $R_A = 20$ mm Hg $\cdot$ l^{-1} $\cdot$ min. At a normal cardiac output (5,000 ml/min) and a normal blood volume (5,600 ml) what would be this person's arterial pressure (P_A)?

    Solution:

    (a) This is a tricky question.

(b) The arterial pressure can be approximated (Chap. 6) by an application of the Poiseuille equation (Eq. 5) as follows

$$P_A = R_A \dot{Q} + P_V$$

P_V = the venous pressure. If we assume that P_V = 0, then

$$P_A = R_A \dot{Q} = \underset{\dfrac{\text{mm Hg (l/min)}}{\text{(l/min)}}}{20} \cdot 5 = 100 \text{ mm Hg}$$

(c) Yet we know that the arterial compliance is 2.57 $ml \cdot kg^{-1} \cdot mm\ Hg^{-1}$ which means that the arterial blood volume, at an arterial blood pressure of 100 mm Hg, must be

$$\underset{\dfrac{\text{(ml/kg)}\quad\text{kg}\quad\text{mm Hg}}{\text{mm Hg}}}{2.57 \cdot 70 \cdot 100} \quad \text{or } 17,990 \text{ ml}$$

This represents a volume in excess of that present (5,000 ml) of 12,990 ml.

Answer:
Obviously this represents a ridiculous situation which cannot occur. To maintain the blood pressure imposed by the arterial pressure-flow relationship (R_A and $\dot{Q}$) would necessitate an arterial blood volume far in excess of that available, not to mention the fact that venous volume would quickly be transferred into the arterial system which would reduce to zero venous return and cardiac output.

Comment:
This question points to the necessity of having a venous system of high compliance and an arterial system of low compliance.

16. You are studying the circulation of an anesthetized, paralyzed, and open-chested patient being ventilated with a positive pressure respirator. Assume a linear pressure drop down the circulatory system and a cardiac output linearly related to the difference between mean systemic pressure and right atrial pressure (P_{RA}). The right atrial pressure is maintained at zero (atmospheric pressure). The unstressed volume (V_0) of the circulation is assumed to be at zero; 1,259 ml of blood volume are added to the circulatory system above its unstressed volume. The compliance of the systemic circulation (C_S) is 179 ml/mm Hg. The total peripheral resistance

(TPR) is 20.0 mm Hg·l^{-1}·min, and the resistance to venous return (R$_V$) is 7 percent of TPR.

(A) Calculate control conditions.

(1) What is the mean systemic pressure (P$_{MS}$)?
(2) What is the cardiac output (Q̇)?
(3) What is the arterial pressure (P$_A$)?

Solution:

(a) Recall from Equation 10 that the volume-pressure relationship of the vascular reservoir defines the mean systemic pressure. Thus

$$P_{MS} = \frac{V - V_o}{C_S}, \qquad (10)$$

where $V - V_o$ = blood volume above the unstressed volume. The value of P$_{MS}$ can be found by substituting the appropriate values

$$P_{MS} = \frac{(1259)}{179} = 7.0 \text{ mm Hg}.$$

(b) Cardiac output is simply defined as

$$\dot{Q} = \frac{P_{MS} - P_{RA}}{R_V}.$$

Since R$_V$ = 7 percent of TPR, P$_{MS}$ = 7 mm Hg and P$_{RA}$ = 0.

$$\dot{Q} = \frac{7 - 0}{1.4} = 5.0 \text{ l/min}.$$

(c) The arterial pressure can be obtained (Chap. 6) by an application of the Poiseuille equation (Eq. 5)

$$P_A = (TPR)\dot{Q} + P_{RA}.$$

Therefore

$$P_A = 20.0 \cdot 5 + 0 = 100 \text{ mm Hg}.$$

Answers:
(1) $P_{MS} = 7.0$ mm Hg.
(2) $\dot{Q} = 5.0$ l/min.
(3) $P_A = 100$ mm Hg.
Comment:
The values derived above are normal values for an average 70-kg man.
(B) The blood volume of the circulation system above V_0 is now doubled.
(1) What is P_{MS}?
(2) What is $\dot{Q}$?
(3) What is P_A?
Solution:
The solution to this section is identical to part A, except V = 2,518 ml.
Answers:
(1) 14 mm Hg.
(2) 10 l/min.
(3) 200 mm Hg.
(C) The initial volume of the circulatory system above V_0 is restored, and a slow norepinephrine drip is started. In 20 minutes C_S is found to be ½ its initial value.
(1) What is P_{MS}?
(2) What is $\dot{Q}$?
(3) What is P_A?

Solution:
The solution to this section is identical to part A, except C_S = 89.5 ml/mm Hg.
Answers:
(1) 14 mm Hg.
(2) 10 l/min.
(3) 200 mm Hg.
Comment:
These questions illustrate the basic fact that both the volume and the elastic characteristics of the systemic circulation are determinants of cardiac output.

17. A coronary patient is lying supine in an intensive care unit. Through x-ray examination and cardiac catheterization the physician has the following information: At end expiration, the A-P distance of the patient's lungs = 10 cm, mean pulmonary arterial pressure (P_{PA}) = 25 cm H_2O, alveolar pressure = zero, left atrial pressure (P_{LA}) referred to the bottom of the lung = 13 cm H_2O, right atrial pressure (P_{RA}) = 2 cm H_2O, cardiac output ($\dot{Q}$) = 4 l/min, and mean systemic pressure (P_{MS}) is assumed to be normal at 10 cm H_2O.
(A) The patient breathes spontaneously and at end inspiration both P_{LA} and P_{RA} are found to fall 3 cm H_2O as pulmonary vascular resistance drops 30 percent. The A–P distance of the lung does not change significantly. How much does P_{PA} change at end inspiration?
Solution:
(a) Pulmonary arterial pressure is a function of both pulmonary vascular resistance and cardiac output; therefore, we must determine the quantitative change in each.
(b) From Equation 11 in Chapter 5 we recall

$$\dot{Q} = \frac{P_{MS} - P_{RA}}{R_{VS}}.$$
(11)

(c) At end expiration

$$R_{VS} = \frac{10 - 2}{4} = 2 \text{ cm } H_2O \cdot l^{-1} \cdot min.$$

(d) Assuming R_{VS} and P_{MS} remain constant with respiration, at end inspiration

$$\dot{Q} = \frac{10 - 0}{2} = 5 \; l/min.$$

Note that, although P_{RA} fell 3 cm H_2O, the driving pressure for venous return (and cardiac output) increased only 2 cm H_2O because of collapse of the great veins (see Eq. 12).

(e) Pulmonary vascular resistance can be calculated by

$$PVR = \frac{P_{PA} - P_{PV}}{\dot{Q}} .$$

P_{PV} was selected as the appropriate back pressure for the calculation of PVR because the entire lung was in a zone III condition, i.e. no portion of the lung had a pulmonary venous pressure less than alveolar pressure. Therefore at end expiration

$$PVR = \frac{25 - 13}{4} = 3 \; cm \; H_2O \cdot l^{-1} \cdot min.$$

(f) Since at end inspiration PVR drops 30 percent, $PVR = 2.1$ cm $H_2O \cdot l^{-1} \cdot min$ at end inspiration.

(g) At end inspiration

$$P_{PA} = (PVR)\dot{Q} + P_{PV}$$
$$P_{PA} = (2.1)5 + 10 = 20.50 \; cm \; H_2O.$$

Answer:
In this patient there is no significant change in P_{PA} during a spontaneous breath.
Comment:
During lung inflation the small pulmonary vessels tend to be compressed, but during a spontaneous breath the increase in venous return (and right heart output) largely negates this compression.

(B) The above patient develops pulmonary edema because of the high left atrial pressure. All hemodynamic parameters are the same at end expiration. To assist his ventilation he is placed on a positive pressure ventilator with an end expiratory pressure of 20 cm H_2O. Since air flow through the lungs has stopped at end expiration, we can assume alveolar pressure is equal to 20 cm H_2O. At end inspiration PVR is found to double as both P_{RA} and P_{LA} rise 3 cm H_2O. How much does P_{PA} change at end inspiration?
Solution:

    (a) Since at end expiration the hemodynamic parameters have not changed

$$R_{VS} = 2 \text{ cm } H_2O \cdot l^{-1} \cdot min$$
$$PRV = 3 \text{ cm } H_2O \cdot l^{-1} \cdot min.$$

    (b) At end inspiration

$$\dot{Q} = \frac{10 - 5}{2} = 2.5 \text{ l/min.}$$

    (c) At end inspiration

$$PVR = 6 \text{ cm } H_2O \cdot l^{-1} \cdot min.$$

(d) At end inspiration

$$PVR = (PVR)\dot{Q} + P_A$$
$$P_{PA} + (6)2.5 + 20 = 35 \text{ cm } H_2O.$$

Note that under the conditions of positive pressure ventilation alveolar pressure is greater than pulmonary venous pressure; therefore, the lung is in a zone II condition, and P_A must replace P_{PV} as the back pressure.

Answer:
P_{PA} increases 75 percent during artificial respiration.
Comment:
During lung inflation by positive pressure ventilation the compression of the small pulmonary vessels is manifested as an increase in PVR and an increased back pressure. The increase in PVR is accentuated by the drop in venous return. The net result is an increase in the amount of work the right ventricle has to do and can be associated with harmful consequences, particularly in a patient who has preexisting impairment of right ventricular function.

18. Which of the following changes would be associated with an increase in cardiac output (right atrial pressure = 2 mm Hg). Answer yes or no to each.
(A) Blood transfusion
(B) Decrease in compliance of the venules
(C) Increase in strength of myocardial contraction
(D) Increase in heart rate
(E) External pressure on the abdomen
(F) Going from a supine to a standing position
(G) Standing in a swimming pool with the water up to the umbilicus
(H) Increase in coronary blood flow
(I) Decrease in resistance of veins
Answers:
(A) yes   (B) yes   (C) yes   (D) yes   (E) yes   (F) no
(G) yes   (H) yes   (I) yes

Comments:

(A) The increase in blood volume resulting from a transfusion would increase the mean systemic pressure; therefore, the driving pressure for venous return (and also cardiac output) would be increased.

(B) A decrease in venous compliance would increase the mean systemic pressure; therefore, the driving pressure for venous return (and also cardiac output) would be increased.

(C) A right atrial pressure of 2 mm Hg indicates an atrium distended with blood. Increasing the strength of myocardial contraction would increase the stroke volume, emptying the atrium of blood and lowering its pressure. Cardiac output would increase until right atrial pressure fell to zero and the veins entering the chest collapsed. Thereafter, cardiac output would be limited by systemic factors.

(D) A right atrial pressure of 2 mm Hg indicates an atrium distended with blood. Increasing the heart rate would increase the minute volume pumped by the heart, thereby emptying the atrium of blood and lowering its pressure. Cardiac output would increase until right atrial pressure fell to zero. Thereafter, cardiac output would be limited by systemic factors.

(E) External pressure on the abdomen would act to increase the effective mean systemic pressure; therefore, the driving pressure for venous return (and also cardiac output) would be increased.

(F) Going from a supine to a standing position acts to lower the pressure in the compliant areas of the gut, relative to the right atrium, lowering the effective mean systemic pressure and, therefore, reducing the driving pressure for venous return (and cardiac output).

(G) Water around the abdomen acts as an external pressure on the abdomen, increasing the effective mean systemic pressure; therefore the driving pressure for venous return (and also cardiac output) would be increased.

(H) An increase in coronary blood flow should increase the force of contraction emptying the distended atrium (indicated by an atrial pressure of 2 mm Hg). Cardiac output would increase until right atrial pressure fell to zero and the atrium collapsed. Thereafter the cardiac output would be limited by systemic factors.

(I) A decrease in the venous resistance would directly increase the venous return and, therefore, the cardiac output.

19. Which of the following changes would be associated with an increase in cardiac output (right atrial pressure = 0). Answer yes or no.

(A) Blood transfusion

(B) Decrease in compliance of the venules

(C) Increase in strength of myocardial contraction

(D) Increase in heart rate

(E) External pressure on the abdomen

(F) Going from a supine to a standing position

(G) Standing in a swimming pool with the water up to the umbilicus

(H) Increase in coronary blood flow

(I) Decrease in resistance of veins

Answers:

(A) yes   (B) yes   (C) no   (D) no   (E) yes   (F) no
(G) yes   (H) no   (I) yes

Comments:

(A) The increase in blood volume resulting from a transfusion would increase the mean systemic pressure; therefore, the driving pressure for venous return (and also cardiac output) would be increased.

(B) A decrease in venous compliance would increase the mean systemic pressure; therefore, the driving pressure for venous return (and also cardiac output) would be increased.

(C) Since in this example the right atrium is collapsed (indicated by a right atrial pressure of zero) cardiac output is determined exclusively by systemic factors; therefore, increasing myocardial contraction would have no effect on cardiac output.

(D) Since in this example the right atrium is collapsed (indicated by a right atrial pressure of zero) cardiac output is determined exclusively by systemic factors; therefore, increasing heart rate would have no effect on cardiac output.

(E) External pressure on the abdomen would act to increase the effective mean systemic pressure; therefore, the driving pressure for venous return (and also cardiac output) would be increased.

(F) Going from a supine to a standing position acts to lower the pressure, relative to the right atrium, in the compliant areas of the gut, lowering the effective mean systemic pressure and, therefore, reducing the driving pressure for venous return (and cardiac output).

(G) Water around the abdomen acts as an external pressure

on the abdomen, increasing the effective mean systemic pressure; therefore, the driving pressure for venous return (and also cardiac output) would be increased.

(H) Since in this example the right atrium is collapsed (indicated by a right atrial pressure of zero) cardiac output is determined exclusively by systemic factors; therefore, an increase in coronary blood flow would have no effect on cardiac output.

(I) A decrease in the venous resistance would directly increase the venous return and, therefore, the cardiac output.

15

Study Questions for Section III

20. Assume that the relationship between static pleural pressure (P_{PL}) (during very slow breathing) and lung volume is linear, both during spontaneous breathing and during relaxation. Let the functional residual capacity (FRC) be 3,000 ml and P_{PL} at FRC $= -5$ cm H_2O. Lung volume is increased by 1,000 ml spontaneously, and P_{PL} is found to be -10 cm H_2O. Keeping the lung volume constant at 4,000 ml, all respiratory muscles are relaxed and P_{PL} is found to be -1 cm H_2O.

(A) Paralyze the respiratory muscles and assume no change in the properties of the lungs and thorax and assume that FRC remains the same. Inflate the lungs by positive pressure at the mouth to 3,500 ml (i.e. volume increased by 500 ml).

(1) What is the transpulmonary pressure (P_{TP})?

(2) What is the tracheal pressure (P_T)?

(3) What is the P_{PL}?

Solution: Figure 50.

(a) To solve this problem graphically construct volume and pressure coordinants with volume on the ordinate and pressure on the abscissa. Let FRC be 3,000 ml at the origin of the graph. Allow positive pressures to represent transpulmonary and tracheal pressures, and allow negative pressures to represent pleural pressures.

(b) Construct a compliance curve of the lung as follows. We know that when the patient is breathing spontaneously very slowly, the pleural pressure at 3,000 ml (FRC) is -5 cm H_2O and at 4,000 is -10 cm H_2O. We should also know (although not given in

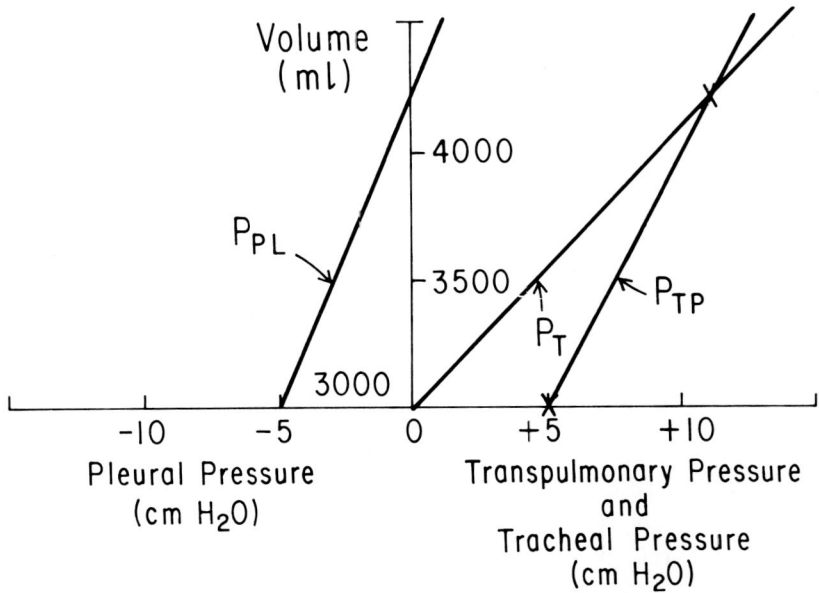

Fig. 50. Graphic solution to Question 20(A).

the question) that during a very slow spontaneous breath alveolar pressure (P_A) remains essentially zero (atmospheric pressure). Therefore, the transpulmonary pressure ($P_A - P_{PL}$) is +5 cm H_2O at 3,000 ml and +10 cm H_2O at 4,000 ml. Connecting these points on the graph gives the compliance curve of the lung.

(c) Construct a compliance curve of the chest wall as follows. We know that at 3,000 ml (FRC) the pleural pressure is −5 cm H_2O and that at 4,000 ml, when the muscles of respiration are relaxed, the pleural pressure is −1 cm H_2O. Connecting these two relaxation points gives the compliance curve of the chest wall.

(d) Construct a series compliance curve of the lung plus chest wall. We know that at FRC (3,000 ml) the tracheal pressure must be zero. We also know that when the thorax is at its unstressed volume ($P_{PL} = 0$) positive pressure applied to the trachea must equal the transpulmonary pressure (i.e. to overcome only the inward elastic recoil of the lungs, because the chest wall at this point is recoiling neither in the inward nor outward direction). Connecting these two points gives the series compliance curve of the lung plus chest wall.

(e) Transpulmonary, tracheal, and pleural pressure can now be read directly from the appropriate compliance curve.

Answers:

(1) $P_{TP} = 7.5$ cm H_2O.

(2) $P_T = 4.5$ cm H_2O.

(3) $P_{PL} = -3.0$ cm H_2O.

(B) While the respiratory muscles were paralyzed, a sufficient amount of negative pressure was applied at the mouth to bring the P_{TP} to 0 cm H_2O.

(1) What was the lung volume?

(2) What was the P_T?

(3) What was the P_{PL}?

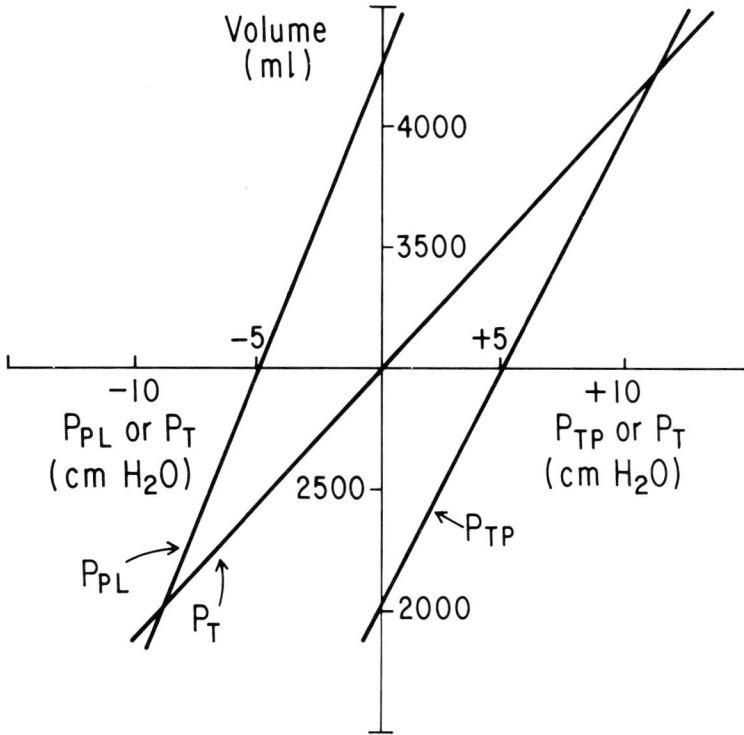

Fig. 51. Graphic solution to Question 20(B).

Solution: Figure 51.

(a) Extend to a lower lung volume all three compliance curves constructed in Figure 50. The lung volume at $P_{TP} = 0$ cm H_2O can now be read from the lung compliance curve.

(b) Read P_T and P_{PL} from the appropriate curves.

Answers:

(1) 2000 ml.

(2) -9.0 cm H_2O.

(3) -9.0 cm H_2O.

(C) The individual whose lungs were discussed above developed lung disease. The thorax was unaffected. It was found that the lung volume at $P_{TP} = 0$ was one-half what it was originally at $P_{TP} = 0$ and that the P_{TP} during spontaneous breathing (very slow breathing) was $+10$ cm H_2O when the lung volume was 2,000 ml.

(1) What was the FRC?

(2) What was P_{PL} at FRC?

(3) What was the P_{PL} during spontaneous breathing at the end of a slow inspiration which increased lung volume by 1,000 ml above FRC?

(4) What kind of change in the lungs could have resulted in these findings?

Solution: Figure 52.

(a) Since the thorax was unaffected the compliance curve of the chest wall is unchanged.

(b) We know that originally the lung volume (V_L) at $P_{TP} = 0$ was 2,000 ml; therefore, if it is now one-half its original value it must be 1,000 ml.

(c) Construct a new compliance curve of the lung by connecting the points 1,000 ml V_L and 10 cm H_2O P_{TP}.

(d) FRC can be obtained by finding the volume where P_{PL} is equal but opposite P_{TP}.

(e) P_{PL} at FRC can now be read from the chest wall compliance curve.

(f) Recall that pleural pressure at the end of a slow spontaneous breath is equal but opposite to the transpulmonary pressure since alveolar pressure is zero.

Answers:

(1) 1,940 ml.

(2) -9.25 cm H_2O.

(3) -19.75 cm H_2O.

(4) Interstitial or alveolar fibrosis.

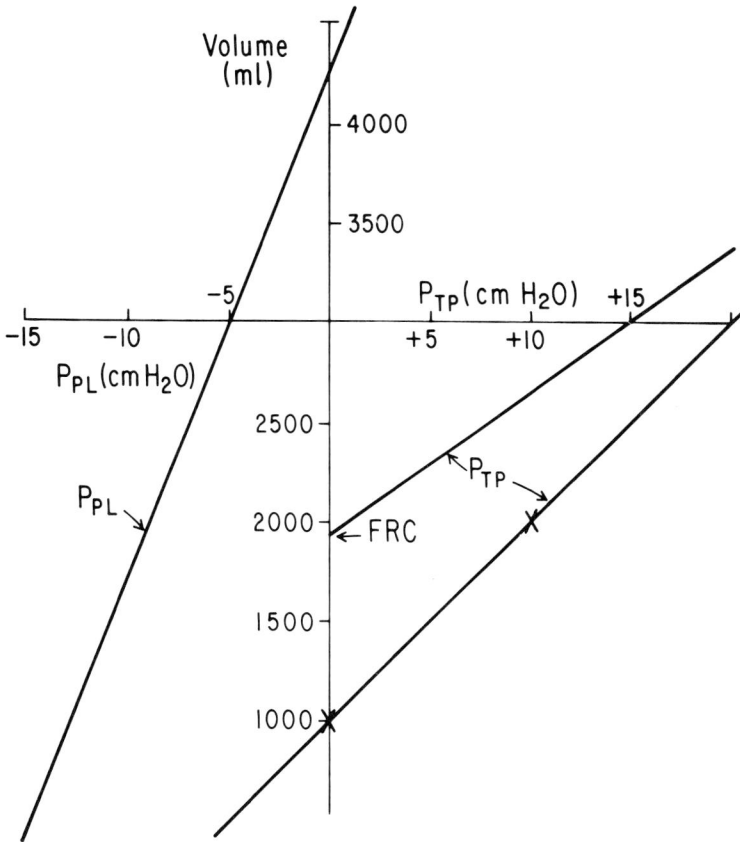

Fig. 52.   Graphic solution to Question 20(C).

21. The physician in a pulmonary function laboratory finds that a patient has a functional residual capacity of 2,400 ml. As he takes a breath from FRC (spontaneous inspiration), his esophageal pressure falls 4 cm H_2O as 800 ml are inhaled. What is the lung compliance?

Solution:

   (a) Lung compliance is $\Delta V/\Delta P_{TP}$.

   (b) $\Delta V = 800$ ml.

   (c) $\Delta P_{TP} = 4$ cm H_2O.

Answer:

200 ml/cm H_2O.

22. During a slow spontaneous breath in a patient the pleural pressure changed from -5 cm H_2O at end expiration to -10 cm H_2O at end inspiration. During artificial respiration with the same tidal volume as during spontaneous respiration (muscle of respiration relaxed), the pleural pressure changed from -5 cm H_2O at end expiration to -1 cm H_2O at end inspiration.

(A) Was the compliance of the thorax greater than the compliance of the lungs?

(B) What was the tracheal pressure (P_T) at end inspiration during artificial respiration?

(C) What was the tracheal pressure at the end of a passive expiration?

Solution:

(a) During a slow spontaneous breath alveolar pressure is essentially zero; therefore $P_{PL} = P_{TP} = 5$ cm H_2O.

(b) During artificial respiration, with the muscles of respiration relaxed, the changes in pleural pressure (4 cm H_2O) can be used to assess chest wall compliance.

(c) Lung compliance is $\Delta V/\Delta P_{TP}$; chest wall compliance is $\Delta V/\Delta P_{PL}$.

(d) The transpulmonary pressure at end inspiration must be the same regardless of whether the breath was spontaneous or artificial because the lung volume was the same.

(e) P_{TP} at end inspiration, therefore, must equal 5 cm H_2O.

(f) $P_T = P_{TP} + P_{PL}$.

Answers:

(A) No.

(B) 4 cm H_2O.

(C) Atmospheric pressure.

23. Work, defined as the product of pressure times volume, must be done if breathing is to occur. This *work of breathing* results not only from energy expended by the respiratory muscles to expand the lungs but also to overcome airway resistance, R_{AW}. Define by use of a pressure-volume diagram:

(A) The work of inspiration from FRC to overcome lung recoil.

(B) The work to overcome R_{AW} during inspiration from FRC.

(C) The energy stored in the elastic tissues of the lung to overcome R_{AW} during expiration to FRC.

(D) The total work of inspiration from FRC to overcome recoil of lung plus R_{AW}.

(E) The energy stored in the chest wall during inspiration.

(F) Net inspiratory work of respiratory system from FRC.

Solution: Figure 53.

    (a) Construct volume and pressure coordinates with volume on the ordinate, and pleural pressure (P_{PL}) on the abscissa. Let FRC and zero P_{PL} be at the origin of the graph.

    (b) On these coordinants place a hypothetical chest wall compliance curve in the normal position.

    (c) Plot a hypothetical lung compliance curve as lung volume against pleural pressure, the assumption being the alveolar pressure is zero. This curve will be a mirror image of the usual compliance curve (V_L/P_{TP}).

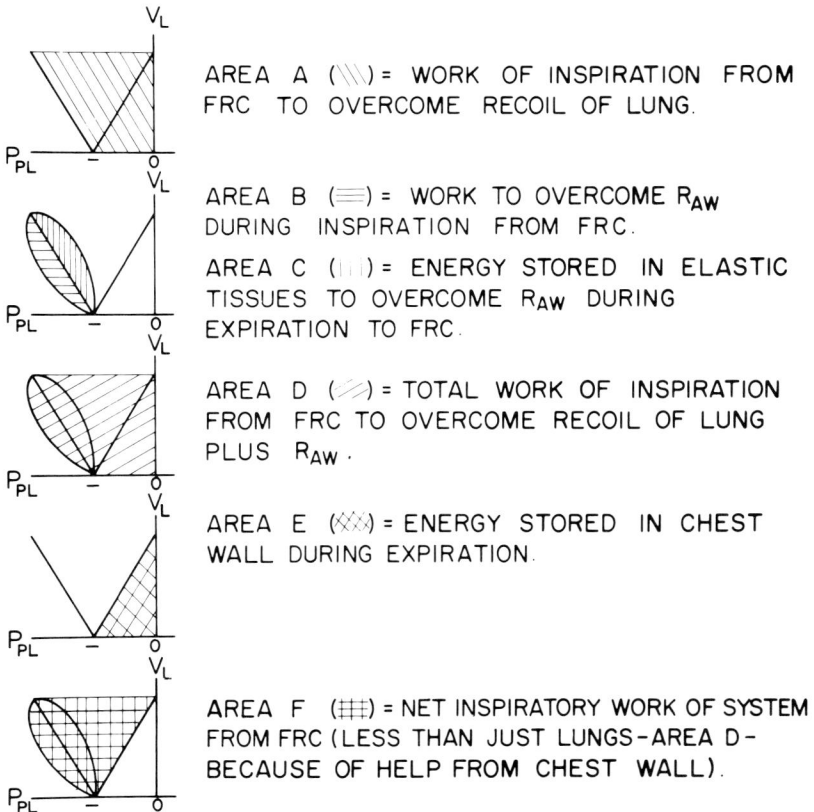

AREA A ($\backslash\backslash\backslash$) = WORK OF INSPIRATION FROM FRC TO OVERCOME RECOIL OF LUNG.

AREA B ($\equiv$) = WORK TO OVERCOME R_{AW} DURING INSPIRATION FROM FRC.

AREA C ($|||$) = ENERGY STORED IN ELASTIC TISSUES TO OVERCOME R_{AW} DURING EXPIRATION TO FRC.

AREA D ($/\!/$) = TOTAL WORK OF INSPIRATION FROM FRC TO OVERCOME RECOIL OF LUNG PLUS R_{AW}.

AREA E ($\times\!\times$) = ENERGY STORED IN CHEST WALL DURING EXPIRATION.

AREA F ($\#\#$) = NET INSPIRATORY WORK OF SYSTEM FROM FRC (LESS THAN JUST LUNGS – AREA D – BECAUSE OF HELP FROM CHEST WALL).

Fig. 53. Solution to Question 23.

Answer:
See Figure 53.

24. The pulmonary function of a 20-year-old college student was studied. His isovolume pressure-flow curve at a lung volume of 3 liters was determined. His expiratory flow increased linearly from zero to 300 l/min as the pressure drop between alveoli and mouth (ΔP) increased from zero to 20 cm H_2O (ΔP′). Increasing ΔP above ΔP′ did not increase maximum expiratory flow ($\dot{V}_{E\ max}$). Calculate this individual's total airway resistance.
Solution:
   (a) Recall that $\dot{V}_{E\ max}$ in an isovolume pressure-flow curve is due to airway collapse. Therefore the reciprocal of the slope of the isovolume pressure-flow curve, up to but not beyond the point where airway collapse occurs, can be used to calculate airway resistance.
   (b)

$$R_{AW} = \frac{\Delta P'}{\dot{V}_{E\ max}} = \frac{20 \text{ cm } H_2O}{300 \text{ l/min}} = .067 \text{ cm } H_2O \cdot l^{-1} \cdot min.$$

Answer:
.067 cm $H_2O \cdot l^{-1} \cdot$ min.

25. Thirty years later this same individual (Question 24) develops bronchitis and returns to the pulmonary function laboratory for another pulmonary function study. At age 50 this patient is able to develop a $\dot{V}_{E\ max}$ of only 200 l/min as ΔP increased to 20 cm H_2O. How much has this patient's airway resistance increased?
Solution:

$$R_{AW} = \frac{\Delta P'}{\dot{V}_{E\ max}} = \frac{20 \text{ cm } H_2O}{200 \text{ l/min}} = .1 \text{ cm } H_2O \cdot l^{-1} \cdot min.$$

Answer:
49 percent.

26. A few years later the same patient develops asthma. He now achieves a $\dot{V}_{E\ max}$ of 100 l/min with a ΔP of 10 cm H_2O. What is his airway resistance now?
    Solution:

$$R_{AW} = \frac{\Delta P'}{\dot{V}_{E\ max}} = \frac{10\ cm\ H_2O}{100\ l/min} = .1\ cm\ H_2O \cdot l^{-1} \cdot min.$$

Answer:
The same as before (Question 24).
Comment:
If the resistance to air flow did not change, then the reduction in $\dot{V}_{E\ max}$ must have come from an increase in the effective back pressure to flow, i.e. the strength of airway collapse. The analysis of an isovolume pressure-flow curve in just this way has led to the hypothesis that an increase in bronchial smooth muscle tone, such as occurs in asthma, results in an increase in the effective back pressure to expiratory flow in much the same way that an increase in arterial smooth muscle tone increases the effective arterial back pressure. The result of this analysis is the postulation that reversible airway obstruction, such as asthma, results from an increase in bronchial smooth muscle tone in the large collapsible airways, increasing the back pressure, whereas irreversible airway obstruction, such as emphysema, is a manifestation of a permanent increase in the airway resistance in the small airways between the alveoli and the collapsible portion of the large airways. This concept was developed in Chapter 12.

SECTION V: APPENDICES

Appendix I: The Language

The symbols used by physiologists have always been confusing. The reason is simple: different physiologists used different symbols to represent the same parameter. Fortunately in 1950 a group of physiologists got together and agreed to a standard set of symbols and abbreviations. This reduced the confusion tremendously but did not eliminate it. For example, some physiologists will use the symbol V to mean blood volume while others will use Q. In preparing this text an attempt was made to use the symbols which are in the most common use today. Those for gases and blood were adapted by the 1950 convention (Fed. Proc., 9:602–605, 1950) and are listed below. A dash (—) above a symbol indicates a mean value, while a dot ($\cdot$) above a symbol means a time derivative.

For Gases

Primary symbols (capital letters)

V = gas volume

$\dot{V}$ = gas flow (volume/time)

P = gas pressure

$\bar{P}$ = mean gas pressure

Secondary symbols (small capital letters, slightly below the primary symbols)

ɪ = inspiratory gas

ᴇ = expiratory gas

ᴀ = alveolar gas

ʙ = barometric

For Blood

Primary symbols (capital letters)

Q = blood volume

$\dot{Q}$ = blood flow (volume/time)

149

Secondary symbols (small letters)

    a = arterial blood

    v = venous blood

    c = capillary blood

        Other Commonly Used Symbols

    P = blood pressure

    $\bar{P}$ = mean blood pressure

    R = resistance

  C.O. = cardiac output

  V.R. = venous return

    F = fraction of cardiac output

 A.W. = airway

Some common examples:

    $\bar{P}_a$ = mean arterial blood pressure

    R_a = arterial resistance

    R_v = venous resistance

    $\dot{V}_I$ = inspiratory air flow

    $\dot{V}_E$ = expiratory air flow

Appendix II: Hemodynamics

Hydraulics is the study of fluids in motion. Since Newton's second law of motion ($F = m \times a$) must be obeyed by each and every particle of fluid, hydraulics can become one of the most complex branches of mechanics if the proper conditions are not fulfilled. If the conditions are fulfilled, the flow of fluid is of a relatively simple type called streamline or steady flow, and equations of motion may be relatively simply derived. In streamline flow every particle of fluid passing a particular point follows exactly the same path as the preceding particles which passed that same point. These paths are called lines of flow or streamlines. The fundamental relationships of hydraulics are defined by the *Bernoulli equation* which relates pressure, velocity, and elevation at points along the streamline. The Bernoulli equation is essentially an application of the principle of conservation of energy to fluid flow (i.e. the work done on a particle of fluid must equal the sum of its initial and final energies).

For the moment let us consider the flow through a rigid conduit of a nonviscous, incompressible fluid. Figure 54 represents a portion of such a conduit. Let us follow a small bolus of fluid, indicated by shading, as it passes from one point to another along the conduit.

Let h_1 be the elevation of the first point above some reference level, v_1 the velocity at that point, A_1 the cross-sectional area of the conduit, and P_1 the pressure. All of these quantities may vary from point to point, and h_2, v_2, A_2, and P_2 are their values at a second point.

Since the fluid is under pressure at all points, inward forces shown by the heavy arrows are exerted against both faces of the bolus. As the element moves from point one to point two, work is

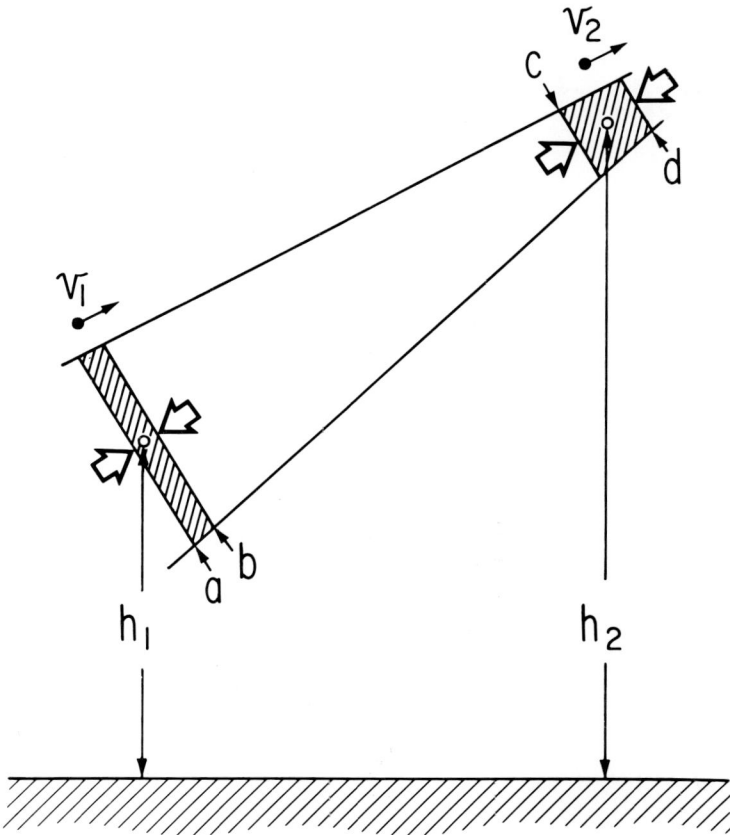

Fig. 54. Portion of a rigid conduit through which flows a nonviscous incompressible fluid. See text for details.

done *on* it by the force acting on its left face, and work is done *by* it against the force acting on its right face. The net work done on the bolus (i.e. difference between these quantities) equals the gain in its kinetic and potential energy.

If A represents the cross-sectional area of the conduit at any point, and P the corresponding pressure, the force against a face of the bolus at any point is P × A. The work done *on* the element in the motion in the diagram is

$$_a\int^c Fds = {_a}\int^c P\,Ads,$$

where ds is any short distance measured along the tube, and the limits are from A to C, since these are the initial and final positions of the left face. This integral may be written

$$\int_a^c P\,A\,ds = \int_a^b P\,A\,ds + \int_b^c P\,A\,ds.$$

Similarly, the work done *by* the element in its motion is

$$\int_b^d P\,A\,ds = \int_b^c P\,A\,ds + \int_c^d P\,A\,ds.$$

The net work done on the element is

$$\int_a^b P\,A\,ds + \int_b^c P\,A\,ds - \int_b^c P\,A\,ds - \int_c^d P\,A\,ds =$$

$$\int_a^b P\,A\,ds - \int_c^d P\,A\,ds.$$

The distances from A to B and from C to D are sufficiently small so that the pressures and areas may be considered constant along these limits. Therefore

$$\int_a^b P\,A\,ds = P_1\,A_1\,\Delta S_1 \text{ and}$$

$$\int_c^d P\,A\,ds = P_2\,A_2\,\Delta S_2.$$

However, $A_1\Delta S_1 = A_2\Delta S_2 = V$, where V is the volume of the bolus. Hence

$$\text{net work} = (P_1 - P_2)\ V. \tag{30}$$

Let ρ be the density of the liquid and m be the mass of the bolus. Then $V = \dfrac{m}{\rho}$, and Equation 30 becomes

$$\text{net work} = (P_1 - P_2)\ \frac{m}{\rho}\ .$$

We now equate the net work on the element to the sum of the increases in its kinetic and potential energy

$$(P_1 - P_2)\ \frac{m}{\rho} = (\ \frac{1}{2}\ mv_2^2 - \frac{1}{2}\ mv_1^2\ ) + (mgh_2 - mgh_1).$$

Rearranging yields

$$(P_1 - P_2)\ \frac{m}{\rho} + (\ \frac{1}{2}\ mv_1^2 + mgh_1) = (\ \frac{1}{2}\ mv_2^2 + mgh_2). \tag{31}$$

Equation 31 states that the work done on the bolus plus the initial energy of the bolus must equal the final energy of the bolus. Thus, energy has been conserved. After cancelling m and rearranging terms, we obtain

$$P_1 + \frac{1}{2} \rho v_1^2 + \rho g h_1 = P_2 + \frac{1}{2} \rho v_2^2 + \rho g h_2. \qquad (32)$$

Equation 32 states that, as a nonviscous bolus flows from point one to point two, the total energy at point one will equal the total energy at point two. Since the subscripts 1 and 2 referred to any two points along the conduit we may write

$$P + \frac{1}{2} \rho v^2 + \rho g h = \text{constant total fluid energy.} \quad (33)$$

Either Equation 32 or Equation 33 is known as the Bernoulli equation. Note that P is the absolute (not measured) pressure and must be in dynes per square centimeter (not mm Hg), and the density must be expressed in grams per cubic centimeter. Thus, assuming the fluid perfusing our conduit is nonviscous, the total fluid energy at any two points will be the same. This, however, is unrealistic because most fluids, especially those found in biologic systems, such as blood, possess at least some degree of viscosity. Viscosity may be thought of as the internal friction of a fluid. Because of viscosity, a force must be exerted to cause one layer of fluid to slide past another or to slide past the surface of a conduit. Since a force must be exerted to overcome the internal friction of the fluid (the viscosity) the total fluid energy at two points along the conduit in reality cannot be the same, for the fluid energy at the upstream end must be greater than the fluid energy at the downstream end by an amount necessary to overcome the internal friction. That is, the total fluid energy at point two, E_{T2}, must equal the total fluid energy at point one, E_{T1}, minus some amounts of energy due to frictional losses, E_f. This is symbolized by

$$E_{T2} = E_{T1} - E_f. \qquad (34)$$

This does not mean that energy has been destroyed, since it is found that heat is developed whenever friction forces are present and it can be shown by measuring this heat that it is exactly equivalent to the decrease in total fluid energy; hence, the work done against friction, E_f, is the same as energy converted to heat. (Note: the total energy of any single point for a viscous fluid can still be described by Equation 33; however, the total energy at point two will be less than that at point one by an amount equal to the energy lost to friction.) The force, F_f, that is necessary to overcome the internal friction of a fluid has been found experimentally to be proportional to the wall area of a conduit, A, and the gradient of velocity which occurs at right angles to the direction of flow, $\frac{dv}{dr}$, where dv is a small difference in velocity between two points and dr is a small difference in radius between these two points. This relationship is expressed as

$$F_f = \eta A \frac{dv}{dr}.\qquad(35)$$

The proportionality constant is called the *coefficient of viscosity*, or simply the *viscosity*. The unit of viscosity is that of force times distance divided by area times velocity, or, in the cgs system, 1 dyne·sec/cm². A viscosity of 1 dyne·sec/cm² is called a *poise*. Small viscosities are usually expressed in *centipoises* (1 cp$=10^{-2}$ poise). With this quantitative expression for viscosity, we are now in a position to modify the Bernoulli equation to derive an expression which adequately and realistically relates the driving energy for flow to the resulting flow. Consider a rigid, horizontal conduit of internal radius, r, and length, L. Liquid is flowing from point one to point two. Applying Equation 34, we obtain the following relationship for the difference in total fluid energy between point one and point two:

$$P_2 + \frac{1}{2}\rho v_2^2 + \rho g h_2 = P_1 + \frac{1}{2}\rho v_1^2 + \rho g h_1 - E_f.\qquad(36)$$

Since the conduit is horizontal and of constant radius ($r_1 = r_2$ and $h_1 = h_2$), the kinetic energy and hydrostatic potential energy terms cancel from Equation 36. Therefore, the equation reduces to the following expression, which states that the difference in pressure energy between point one and point two is equal to the energy lost due to friction, thus

$$(P_1 - P_2) = E_f.$$

If these energy terms are now expressed as forces, the driving force is

$$(P_1 - P_2)\pi r^2.$$

(Pressure equals force per unit area; therefore, force equals pressure times area.) The viscous force from Equation 35 is

$$F_F = -\eta A \frac{dv}{dr} = -\eta 2\pi r L \frac{dv}{dr}$$

where the minus sign is introduced since v decreases as r increases. That is, the velocity in the center of the tube is the greatest and the velocity at the liquid-surface junction is the least. Equating these forces, we find

$$-\frac{dv}{dr} = (P_1 - P_2)\frac{r}{2\eta L}$$

$$-dv = \frac{P_1 - P_2}{2\eta L} r dr.$$

Integration of this equation gives

$$-v = \frac{P_1 - P_2}{4\eta L} r^2 + C.$$

Let R = complete radius of the tube. Since v = O when r = R

$$-C = \frac{P_1 - P_2}{4\eta L} R^2$$

and therefore

$$v = \frac{P_1 - P_2}{4\eta L} (R^2 - r^2)$$

which is the equation for a parabola. Since the discharge rate, $\dot{Q}$, is

$$d\dot{Q} = vdA = \frac{P_1 - P_2}{4\eta L} (R^2 - r^2) \times 2\pi rdr$$

and

$$\dot{Q} = \int_o^R d\dot{Q} = 2\pi \frac{(P_1 - P_2)}{4\eta L} \int_o^R (R^2 - r^2)\, rdr \qquad (37)$$

$$\dot{Q} = \frac{\pi R^4}{8\eta L} (P_1 - P_2).$$

Equation 37 is known as *Poiseuille's law*. Since capital R is generally used to denote the quantity known as resistance to flow (see below), R from Equation 37 is generally replaced with small r, used to denote the radius. Rearranging the equation, we have

$$\frac{P_1 - P_2}{\dot{Q}} = \frac{8\eta L}{\pi r^4}.$$

Thus the ratio of the total pressure drop of flow is proportional to the viscosity and the length and inversely proportional to the fourth power of the radius. The quantity $\frac{8\eta L}{\pi r^4}$ is generally referred to as the *resistance to flow*, R, because it represents those factors which tend to retard flow. In the cgs system the unit for resistance is dynes·sec/cm^5, pressure being expressed as dynes/sq cm and flow in cm^3/sec.

This simple relationship has been the foundation on which modern hemodynamics is based. Since in most vascular systems the length remains constant and at normal rates of flow the viscosity also remains constant, a change in the resistance is generally interpreted as a change in the vessel's diameter (2r). An increasing diameter results in the fall of vascular resistance and a decreasing diameter in an increase in the vascular resistance. It should be emphasized at this point that these relationships hold only for streamline (steady) flow. The applicability of Poiseuille's law was discussed for both rigid and collapsible conduits in Chapter 4.

References

1. Agostoni, E. and Mead, J.: Statics of the respiratory system. *Handbook of Physiology*, Section 3, Volume I, pp. 387–410, 1964.
2. Bader, H.: The anatomy and physiology of the vascular wall. *Handbook of Physiology*, Section 2, Chapter 26, pp. 865–889, 1963.
3. Bartlestone, H. J.: Role of the veins in venous return. Circ. Res., *8*:1059–1076, 1960.
4. Bates, D. V., Macklem, P. T. and Christie, R. V.: *Respiratory Function in Disease*. Philadelphia, W. B. Saunders, 1971.
5. Bernard, C.: *Lecons sur les Phénoménes de la Vie Communes aux Animaux et aux Végétaux*. Paris, B. Bailliere et Fils, 1879.
6. Burton, A. C.: Relation of structure to function of the tissues of the wall of blood vessels. Physiol. Rev., *34*(4):619–642, 1954.
7. Burton, A. C.: On the physical equilibrium of small blood vessels. Am. J. Physiol., *164*:319–329, 1951.
8. Caldini, P., Permutt, S., Waddell, J. A. and Riley, R. L.: Effect of epinephrine on pressure, flow, and volume relationships in the systemic circulation of the dog. Circ. Res., *34*:606–623, 1974.
9. Cannon, W. B.: Organization for physiological homeostasis. Physiol. Rev., *9*:399–431, 1929.
10. Cherniak, R. M., Cherniack, L. and Naimark, A.: *Respiration in Health and Disease*, 2nd ed. Philadelphia, W. B. Saunders, 1972.
11. Drees, J. A. and Rothe, C. F.: Reflex venoconstriction and capacity vessel pressure-volume relationships in dogs. Circ. Res., *34*:360–373, 1974.
12. Duomarco, J. L. and Rimini, R.: Energy and hydraulic gradients along systemic veins. Am. J. Physiol., *178*:215–231, 1954.
13. Engelberg, J. and Du Bois, A. B.: Mechanics of pulmonary circulation in isolated rabbit lungs. Am. J. Physiol., *186*:401–414, 1959.
14. Glazier, J. B., Hughes, J. M. B., Maloney, J. E. and West, J. B.: Measurements of capillary dimensions and blood volume in rapidly frozen lungs. J. Appl. Physiol., *26*:65–76, 1969.
15. Gato, M. and Kimoto, Y.: Hysteresis and stress-relaxation of the blood vessels studied by a universal tensile testing instrument. Jpn. J. Physiol., *15*:169–184, 1966.
16. Green, J. F. and Attix, E.: Volume-pressure hysteresis in the peripheral venous system of the dog. Fed. Proc., *33*(3):333, 1974.
17. Green, J. F. and Miller, N. C.: A model describing the response of the circulatory system to acceleration stress. Ann. Biomed. Eng., *1*:455–467, 1973.

161

18. Grodins, F. S.: Some simple principles and complex realities of cardiopulmonary control in exercise. Circ. Res., *20* (Suppl. I):171–178, 1967.
19. Guyton, A. C., Jones, C. E. and Coleman, T. C.: *Circulatory Physiology: Cardiac Output and its Regulation*. Philadelphia, W. B. Saunders, 1973.
20. Holt, J. P.: The collapse factor in the measurement of venous pressure: the flow through collapsible tubes. Am. J. Physiol., *134*:292–299, 1941.
21. Howell, J. B., Permutt, S., Proctor, P. F. and Riley, R. L.: Effect of inflation of the lung on different parts of pulmonary vascular bed. J. Appl. Physiol., *16*:71–75, 1961.
22. Hughes, J. M. B., Glazier, J. B., Maloney, J. E. and West, J. B.: Effect of lung volume on the distribution of pulmonary blood flow in man. Respir. Physiol., *4*:58–72, 1968.
23. Knowlton, F. P. and Starling, E. H.: The influence of variations in temperature and blood pressure on the performance of the isolated mammalian heart. J. Physiol. (London), *64*:206–219, 1912.
24. Krogh, A.: Regulation of the supply of blood to the rigid heart (with a description of a new circulation model). Scand. Arch. Physiol., *27*:227–248, 1912.
25. Maseri, A., Caldini, P., Howard, P., Joshi, R. C., Permutt, S. and Zierler, K. L.: Determinants of pulmonary vascular volume—recruitment versus distensibility. Circ. Res., *31*:218–228, 1972.
26. Milnor, W. R.: Pulmonary hemodynamics. In *Cardiovascular Fluid Dynamics*, Vol. 2 (Bergel, D. H., Ed.). New York, Academic Press, 1972.
27. Permutt, S., Bromberger-Barnea, B. and Bane, H. N.: Alveolar pressure, pulmonary venous pressure, and the vascular waterfall. Med. Thorac., *19*:239–260, 1962.
28. Permutt, S. and Riley, R. L.: Hemodynamics of collapsible vessels with tone: the vascular waterfall. J. Appl. Physiol., *18*:924–932, 1963.
29. Remington, J. W.: The physiology of the aorta and major arteries. *Handbook of Physiology*, Section 2, Chapter 24, pp. 799–837, 1963.
30. Remington, J. W.: Hysteresis loop behavior of the aorta and other extensible tissues. Am. J. Physiol., *180*:83–95, 1955.
31. Rodbard, S.: Flow through collapsible tubes: augmented flow produced by resistance at the outlet. Circulation. *11*:280–291, 1955.
32. Pride, N. B., Permutt, S., Riley, R. L. and Bromberger-Barnea, B.: Determinants of maximal expiratory flow from the lungs. J. Appl. Physiol., *23*:646–662, 1967.
33. Richardson, T. Q., Stallings, J. O. and Guyton, A. C.: Pressure-volume curves in live intact dogs. Am. J. Physiol., *201*:471–474, 1961.
34. Shoukas, A. A. and Sagawa, K.: Total systemic vascular compliance measured as incremental volume-pressure ratio. Circ. Res., *28*:277–289, 1971.
35. Shoukas, A. A. and Sagawa, K.: Control of total systemic vascular capacity by the carotid sinus baroreceptor reflex. Circ. Res., *33*:32–33, 1973.
36. Starling, E. H.: Some points in the pathology of heart disease. Effects of heart failure on the circulation. Lancet, *1*:652–655, 1897.
37. West, J. B.: *Ventilation/Blood Flow and Gas Exchange*. Oxford, Blackwell Scientific Press, 1965.
38. West, J. B. and Dollery, C. T.: Distribution of blood flow and ventilation-perfusion ratio in the lung, measured with radioactive CO_2. J. Appl. Physiol., *15*:405–510, 1960.
39. West, J. B. and Dollery, C. T.: Distribution of blood flow and the pressure-flow relations of the whole lung. J. Appl. Physiol., *20*:175–183, 1965.
40. West, J. B., Dollery, C. T. and Naimark, A.: Distribution of blood flow in isolated lung; relative to vascular and alveolar pressures. J. Appl. Physiol., *19*:713–724, 1964.
41. Whitaker, S.: *Introduction to Fluid Mechanics*. Englewood Cliffs, Prentice-Hall, 1968.

Index